Danger Zone

Unlock the Secrets of Nursing Home
Medical Records and
Protect Your Loved One

Dennis R. Steele
Edward C. Watters III, M.D.

A MemberoftheFamily.net LifeGuide®
Member of the Family LLC
Severna Park, Maryland

Danger Zone
Unlock the Secrets of Nursing Home Medical Records and Protect Your Loved One

To
Mary M. Watters

TABLE OF CONTENTS

PREFACE

If you want to know what a nursing home's staff says it is doing for your loved one, look at the medical records. If you want to find out what is really happening, look under the sheets, breathe deeply through your nose, and talk to the patient. And then document everything you observe.

Not all medical records, also known as charts, are fiction, but at a nursing home they are sometimes written with three things in mind: reimbursement, liability, and government oversight. In some homes, the medical credo of "first, do no harm" to the patient has mutated into a less noble strategy. First: get paid for all services, even if they aren't rendered. Second: don't get caught for omissions or commissions. Third: do no harm to the company (and if time permits, tend to the patient).

To achieve *your* top priority – the best possible care for your loved one – you must play the watchdog, a process that can be time-consuming and physically and emotionally draining. Even if you haven't any specific suspicions, it is wise to keep track of patient records. State reports over a several-year cycle have revealed that the number of nursing homes nationwide causing actual harm to patients exceeds 50 percent. Administrators perform the charade of preparing "corrective action plans," but the recidivism rate of homes causing harm rivals that of inmates returning to prison.

In this book, we show you some tricks nursing homes play to keep you – and government regulators – less than fully informed about patient care. You'll also learn some tips for outmaneuvering such attempts to keep you in the dark. And we'll teach you the handy method of using three-by-five cards to document what you observe. For patients whose situation requires more extensive documentation, in the back of the book we have supplied worksheets that break down the areas and items you need to monitor and we have included charts you can use to perform this task.

Danger Zone contains easy-to-understand, nuts-and-bolts advice to help you make sure those you love receive proper treatment.

You'll learn how to:

- gain access to medical records
- read a medical chart
- document care yourself
- fight for your loved one's rights – and yours
- deal with nursing home staff and administration

The most important thing to remember about corporate nursing homes in particular is that they are businesses. Return on investment is always a major consideration when administrators make decisions – about amenities, staffing, meals, and the therapy to be provided. These decisions greatly affect the quality of care the residents in their homes receive.

❑ ❑ ❑

Here's what sets this book apart from many others that provide advice about nursing home care: most other authors believe that if you get involved and work through the system and play nice, you'll be okay. We certainly believe in getting involved, and playing nice may work at some facilities – there's no sense in taking a confrontational approach if the staff is generally cooperative. But the truth is that at many facilities, you'll just get eaten alive playing nice – and you'll only be playing into the administrators' hands. In the world of for-profit nursing homes, everything boils down to money, and the business model is simple: every expense the facility can avoid means more dollars to the bottom line. If you don't challenge the staff about lapses in care – or don't know how to – the home will have won the game, and your loved one could wind up in the danger zone of long-term care in America.

This book will help you level the playing field.

1
KNOWLEDGE + ACTION = POWER

In 1996, during a routine visit to one of his nursing home patients with a sight-threatening disorder, Dr. Edward C. "Terry" Watters, an ophthalmologist and my partner in MemberoftheFamily.net, noticed that the patient's condition had grown discernibly worse since his last visit. He discovered that his orders for treatment had not been followed, and as he was noting this in the patient's chart, a staff member asked him not to do so because that would "cause problems" for the home – financially and with state reporting agencies. The staff member exhibited no concern for any suffering the patient might be experiencing because of the failure to follow the treatment regimen.

During the course of several visits to this home in Baltimore, Dr. Watters noted in the chart additional times when the prescribed regimen had not been followed and confronted the staff about the problem. Again, no one seemed particularly concerned. The last straw came when Terry was told that his notes had been removed from the chart because they might "raise a red flag" for Maryland state reviewers. Outraged, and convinced that the health of all the patients, not just his, was in jeopardy, Dr. Watters called the state's Department of Health and Mental Hygiene to request an immediate investigation.

When nothing happened, he asked a state senator to contact the department. An emergency survey confirmed that chart falsification had occurred, though in another patient's records. No fines were levied, but administrative punishment was applied. Upon learning that Terry had contacted the state, the home's staff pressured him not to do so again, and an executive at the home's parent corporation circulated a letter stating that Dr. Watters was no longer welcome as a consulting specialist in any of its facilities.

This spurred us to action. We learned how to petition for state and federal reports about nursing homes and how to read them. As we assembled the facts and ran statistical analyses, a bleak picture emerged of understaffing, physical abuse, untreated bedsores, and coldhearted decision-making by home operators and state officials charged with monitoring facilities. Residents were viewed simply as numbers, their sole purpose being to help the corporation turn a profit or, with the states, which foot huge bills for care, to keep expenses to a minimum.

Around the same time he was fighting on behalf of his own patient, Terry learned of the cover-up of a death at the same nursing home in Baltimore. Although some nurses were disciplined, the police and the state medical examiner never investigated the matter. This disregard for the lives of elderly patients further strengthened Terry's resolve to fight for change.

A Mother's Legacy

Terry's zeal to help others unlock the secrets of nursing home practices increased all the more a few years later when his mother, Mary Watters, became a resident at a home in Annapolis, Maryland. During the course of her stay – and in spite of his best efforts to ensure she got proper treatment – he witnessed first-hand how staff and administrators cut corners and attempt to shift responsibility for deficient care onto patients and families. Terry, who had power of attorney and later became the court-appointed guardian of property, along with his sister Pat, who was guardian of person, carefully documented what he had observed about their mother's condition, and he and Pat brought their findings to a lawyer. They got the home's attention, though, sadly, not until their mother had passed away.

Terry's experience as a family member with a loved one in a nursing home is as integral to *Danger Zone* as his experience as a physician. As we began assembling materials for the book, it became clear to him that only by looking at actual medical records could our readers truly grasp the documentation process. To that end we have, with the permission of Pat Watters, included pages from their mother's records. Terry and Pat take great comfort in knowing that their mother, a guidance counselor and teacher, will have as her final legacy teaching others to steer clear of substandard care.

You *Can* Improve Conditions

The e-mails we receive weekly on our site have shown us that conditions generally improve for loved ones when family members learn what to look for and how to ask the right questions. A daughter wrote that she used information from a nursing home's state survey results she accessed on MemberoftheFamily.net to improve conditions for her mother in a North Carolina nursing home. She received a phone call and an apology from the administrator after she printed and posted information from the Web site near her mother's bed. Another woman wrote from Kentucky that after showing her mother data about serious hazards at her nursing home, she was able to convince her mother to transfer to another facility. A woman from New Hampshire followed our instructions about documenting care in writing. After she shared her findings with the home's administrator, the care of her family member improved greatly. A writer from Connecticut learned how to obtain her mother's medical charts and what to do with them after she did so. She used that information to make the Department of Public Health, the ombudsman's office, and the Agency on Aging in her state aware of problems in that home.

Although there are many excellent nursing homes in the United States, government reports we have analyzed show that, on their most recent survey, from 20 to 25 percent of all homes will have been found to have caused actual harm to their patients, placed them in immediate jeopardy, or both. And, as we mentioned earlier, over a several-year period this rate climbs to more than 50 percent.

One reason for these alarming statistics has to do with the nature of for-profit businesses, which the majority of nursing homes in the United States are. No matter how caring their brochures may make them seem, they are businesses run by administrators beholden to the bottom line, a reality that can result in long- and short-term strategies not in a patient's best interest. By learning what to observe at a nursing home, how to read medical charts, and how to spot the omissions and discrepancies in them, you will be able to gauge the quality of care the home is providing.

Armed with this knowledge, you will become a better advocate for your loved one.

– Dennis R. Steele

2
MEDICAL RECORDS

Shortly after a nursing home patient passes through the reception area for the first time, the staff shows tremendous interest. Nurses, doctors, and all sorts of assistants drop by to take notes, create tables and charts, and make database entries. In many homes, this may be the only time the team will appear to be working together. Activity reaches a fever pitch at around 2:30 p.m. You, the family member, may feel comforted by all the visitors and attention. Don't be. The shift change is between 3:00 and 4:00, and you might not see this much hustle and bustle again until the staff is helping you gather your relative's personal property so they can prepare the room for the next occupant.

There is a reason for the initial commotion. Insurance carriers and government regulators assume that everything not documented in writing has not been done. Remember the first two tenets of the nursing home's credo: get paid and don't get caught. The documents you see the staff preparing are designed with these goals in mind. Each group is trying to maximize its own reimbursement while at the same time creating an audit-proof chart – a nice way to say they are playing C-Y-A (as in cover your you-know-what), from both the financial and medical perspectives.

Demand the Complete Record

To document care in a nursing home properly, you need to request access to these records – all of them. The first time you do this, you can be sure you will bring all activity on the floor to a screeching halt. You are about to have your first confrontation, unavoidable when you demand entry into the protected world of facility documentation. Everyone involved knows you aren't just looking to see if they have good handwriting, which for the most part they do not. It is possible, though, to couch your request in a way that won't threaten the staff.

The rules of the game are governed by CFR (Code of Federal Regulations) 42 and by state law, which is usually based on the federal regulations. If you are a legitimate agent acting on behalf of a resident, and are not exceeding your authority, you have a right to review medical records within 24 hours of your request and to purchase copies at the local going rate if you give two working-days' notice. Most homes provide immediate access to records but take the two days to supply the copies.

Records are often scattered so far to the wind that only by expending incredible energy can you obtain a complete picture. A favorite ploy at many facilities is "thinning." To assure that all charts will fit in a standard two-inch binder, the oldest ones may be removed until the dimensions are met. The excess documents are often stored in a location that is less than immediately accessible, requiring an extra, sometimes protracted step when inspectors or anyone else needs to see the entire chart. This pretty much guarantees that the sins of the past will not be discovered in the present or future.

Gaining Access

If you have been designated in writing by the patient as the person to make his or her healthcare decisions, or are a court-appointed legal guardian of the person – necessary to have if you will be responsible for care and other decisions for your loved one – gaining access to records should be very easy. Here is how to phrase your request:

> I need to see the chart because in addition to trying to understand what is happening to Mom, I am unable to pay for any services unless they have been provided. All the bills will be audited against the chart for my report to the court and the attorneys representing my family. I'm sure you understand.

You are likely to be stonewalled with phrases such as "I need to check with my supervisor. She will be in on Monday"; or "It is not our policy to allow family members to see the chart." Or the ever-popular, "If you tell me what you are looking for, I will be glad to get it." Don't give in, though. The first time you ask is the roughest. Making the request becomes easier as the staff understands you are trying to fulfill your fiduciary responsibility.

If you have not been designated as the responsible person for healthcare decisions by either the patient or the court, you will likely have problems gaining access to records. If the patient is still mentally competent, he or she can direct the nursing home to release the medical records to you and the staff will have to comply. If a question of competency arises, though, your request to access records will not be considered until the matter of competency is resolved. An individual who has been judged incompetent cannot authorize power of attorney, and the nursing home could refuse to give you the records. If that happens, you will have to apply for guardianship, an expensive and complicated process. Setting up a durable power of attorney as well as advance directives, which include a living will and the designation of a person to make healthcare decisions, should be done before they are needed.

What's in a Medical Record?

So what are you attempting to gain access to? A medical record has six major components. Once you get past the front sheet, the order may vary but the following information will be found in the record:

- Front, or face, sheet
- Order sheets
- Physician/Progress notes
- Nursing notes
- Consultations
- Laboratory data

3
THE FRONT SHEET

As its name implies, the front sheet (Figure 1) is the first piece of paper in a medical record. Check the front sheet for accuracy. This document contains information such as the patient's name, address, room

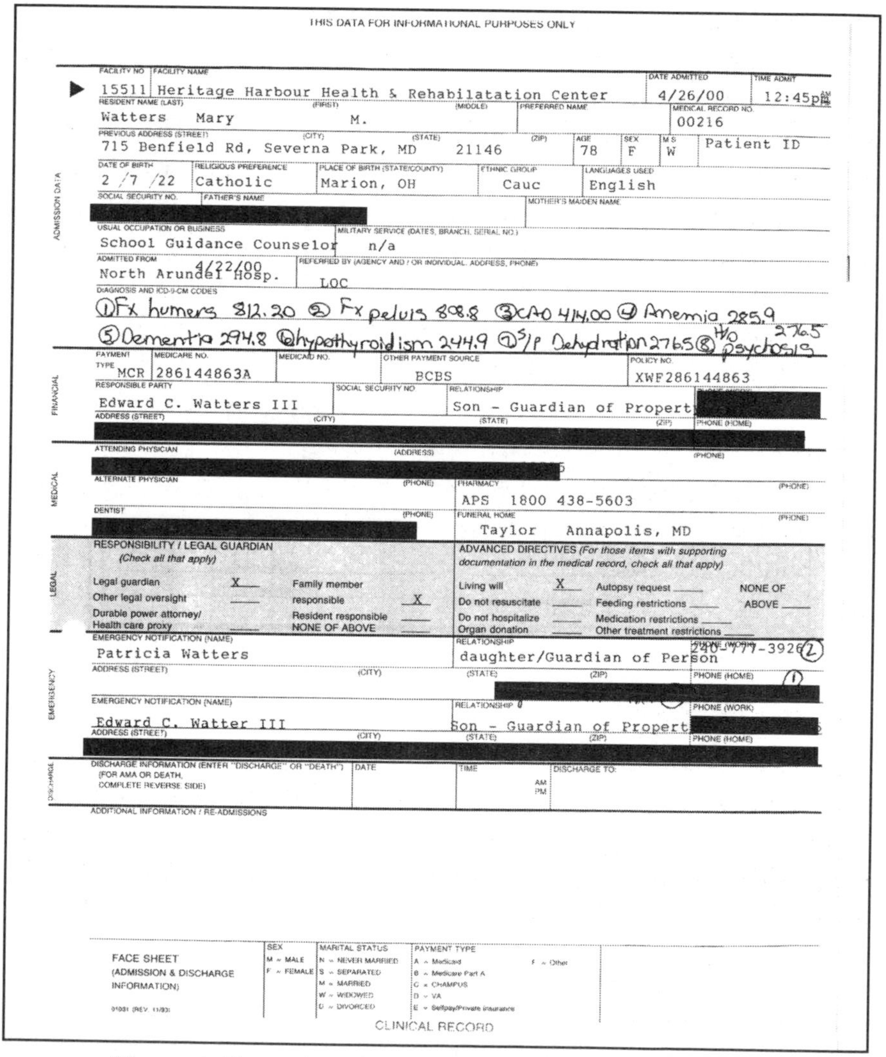

Figure 1: Front sheet, listing critical admission information.

number, attending physician, next of kin, and the person to contact in an emergency. But most important, at least to the nursing home, is the payment information: the name of the insurance company, the insurance I.D. number, any parties financially responsible for the patient, and all billing addresses. In many cases the home may assign various providers, such as an attending physician, alternate physician, dentist, and pharmacy. (You have some choice in these matters, though, as we will explain below.) Any new providers of care or services will review the front sheet. If the financial information is not to their liking, no care or services will occur. Aware of this, facilities often trade access to your loved one, and your money, in return for provider assistance.

For example, though many patients at a facility might qualify for Medicare, a substantial number of them will likely be covered only by Medicaid. Medicare reimbursements follow formulas determined by the federal government. Medicaid reimbursements vary widely from state to state but are nearly always less than Medicare, and therein lies the nursing home's fiscal dilemma: it must provide access to a wide range of services yet somehow find someone willing to work for a substantial discount. The answer is the semi-exclusive contract. If the provider, a physician, for instance, agrees to take all patients irrespective of insurance status, he or she will become the facility's "main provider" and will get first crack at all referrals.

At first glance, having the home's main provider assigned to a family member may seem like a good deal. After all, you won't be getting any bills from the doctor and your loved one will be receiving needed care. Don't be so sure. This arrangement affects the doctor's ability to be an advocate for the patient. Physicians and other providers with many residents in a given home are often loath to risk their financial health for your mom or dad.

If at all possible, your best bet is to retain your family practitioner, who is well known to patient and relatives. Unfortunately, because of financial pressures most such doctors no longer offer the service of visiting patients in nursing homes, though it is worth asking your family practitioner anyway.

4
ORDER SHEETS

A physician or other provider must order all services and treatments, and these must be documented in the medical record. No payments will be made for services rendered without a valid, documented provider request. The order sheet indicates what should be going on with the patient and identifies all the players. Order sheets, though, are not evidence that something was provided to the patient – only that it was ordered. Even doctors fall for this one, so don't feel bad if you do. On a return visit, physicians see that they have written an order, and sometimes misguidedly assume that a staff member's checkmark means the order was executed. The checkmark merely implies that someone on staff has seen the order and it has been transcribed in a different set of records, usually the nurse's notes or the MARS and TARS reports, which are described in the "Nursing Notes" chapter.

The original set of orders when a patient enters a nursing home involves items like activity level, diet, therapy, consultations, code status (such as Do Not Resuscitate), vital signs, and medications. The records normally also indicate the presence or absence of allergies, the medical diagnosis and prognosis, and the level of care to be provided. All the orders are tagged with a date so that the chronology of events is clear. The orders are signed by the physician, and there is some indication that the staff has seen the orders or, in the absence of any orders, that the chart has been reviewed. Order sheets come in three main types: admission orders, physician's orders, and interim orders.

Admission Orders
The first example is an admission order (Figure 2). Get into the habit of checking the patient's name and location on every sheet of paper. Mistakes happen – just don't let them happen to your loved one. You can see the document is well organized. Not just the printed portion on the right side of the page but also the left. The medication and treatment orders are on the left, and ancillary, or nontechnical, ones

are on the right. All the members of the care-giving team are involved: physicians, nurses, therapists, medical assistants, and dieticians.

The right column of the first page, under Ancillary Orders, specifies several things, including the level of care and the discharge plan. The condition of the patient, the diet, the treatment and even recreational activity are also noted. Though all the items may not be familiar, the document appears to be straightforward. But look near the bottom of the page under recreational activities. The box "May not go LOA" is checked in this example. (LOA stands for "leave of absence.") This

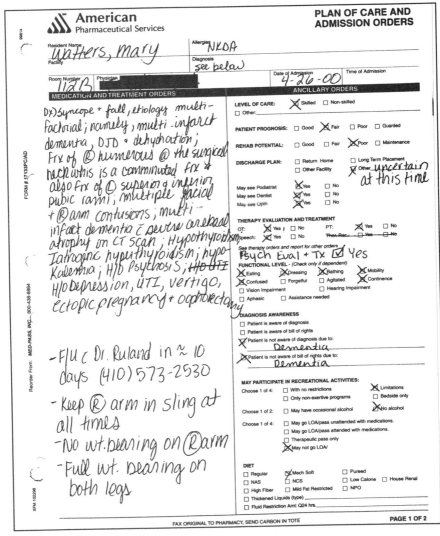

Figure 2a: Admission orders, page 1 of 2.

doesn't mean that the patient is a prisoner or too ill to travel. But under Medicare rules, payment to skilled nursing facilities will not be made if a patient is given LOA status. The patient may go to the doctor's office, no matter how much of an ordeal of driving and waiting that might entail. But he or she cannot go to McDonald's or the park. The theory here is simple – if you happen to be a bureaucrat. Medicare only covers skilled nursing care, and if Mom is "healthy enough" for a simple outing, according to the government she doesn't need skilled care.

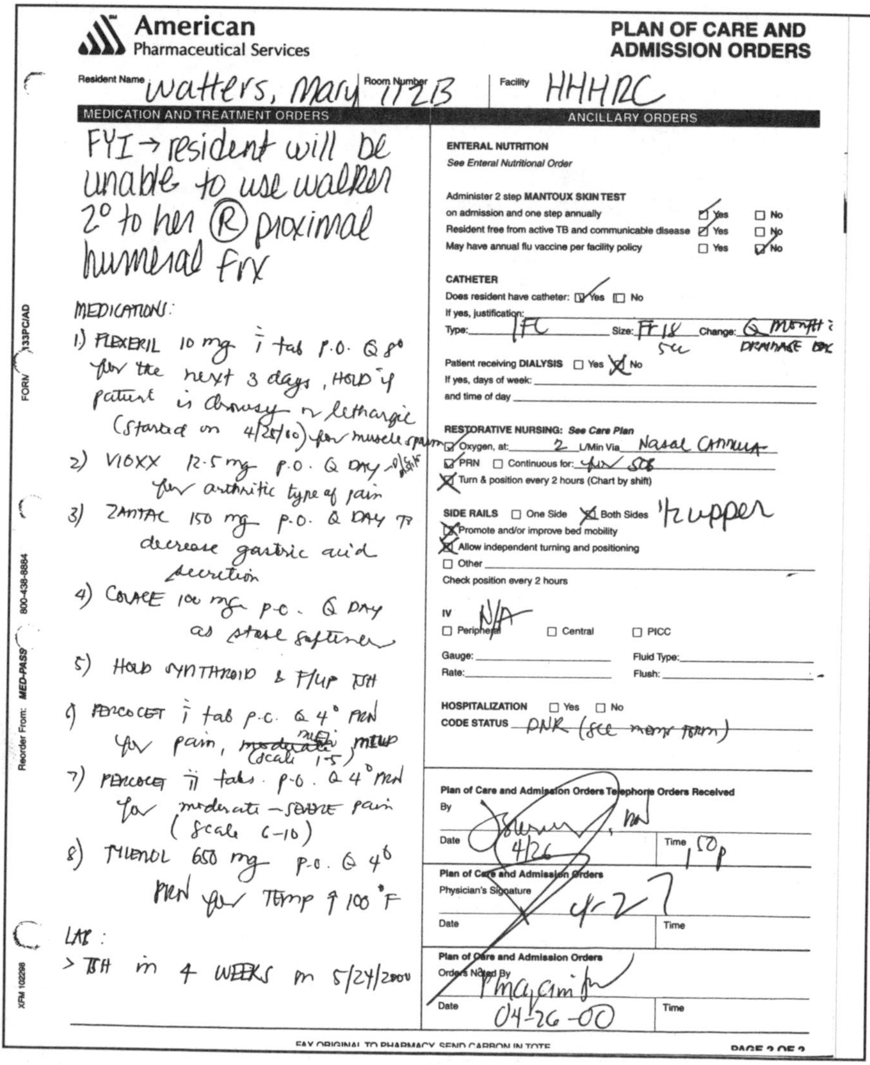

American Pharmaceutical Services

PLAN OF CARE AND ADMISSION ORDERS

Resident Name: Watters, Mary | Room Number: 112B | Facility: HHHRC

MEDICATION AND TREATMENT ORDERS

FYI → resident will be unable to use walker 2° to her Ⓡ proximal humeral frx

MEDICATIONS:

1) FLEXERIL 10 mg i tab P.O. Q 8° for the next 3 days, HOLD if patient is drowsy or lethargic (started on 4/26/10) for muscle spasm
2) VIOXX 12.5 mg P.O. Q DAY for arthritic type of pain
3) ZANTAC 150 mg P.O. Q DAY to decrease gastric acid secretion
4) COLACE 100 mg P.O. Q DAY as stool softener
5) HOLD SYNTHROID & F/UP TSH
6) PERCOCET i tab P.O. Q 4° PRN for pain, ~~moderate~~ mild (scale 1-5)
7) PERCOCET ii tabs P.O. Q 4° PRN for moderate – SEVERE pain (scale 6-10)
8) TYLENOL 650 mg P.O. Q 4° PRN for Temp ↑ 100°F

LAB:
> TSH in 4 WEEKS on 5/24/2000

ANCILLARY ORDERS

ENTERAL NUTRITION
See Enteral Nutritional Order

Administer 2 step MANTOUX SKIN TEST on admission and one step annually ☑ Yes ☐ No
Resident free from active TB and communicable disease ☑ Yes ☐ No
May have annual flu vaccine per facility policy ☐ Yes ☑ No

CATHETER
Does resident have catheter: ☑ Yes ☐ No
If yes, justification:
Type: IFC Size: FF 18 5cc Change: Q month & drainage bag

Patient receiving DIALYSIS ☐ Yes ☒ No
If yes, days of week:
and time of day

RESTORATIVE NURSING: See Care Plan
☑ Oxygen, at: 2 L/Min Via Nasal Cannula
☑ PRN ☐ Continuous for: for SOB
☒ Turn & position every 2 hours (Chart by shift)

SIDE RAILS ☐ One Side ☒ Both Sides ½ upper
☒ Promote and/or improve bed mobility
☒ Allow independent turning and positioning
☐ Other
Check position every 2 hours

IV N/A
☐ Peripheral ☐ Central ☐ PICC
Gauge: Fluid Type:
Rate: Flush:

HOSPITALIZATION ☐ Yes ☐ No
CODE STATUS DNR (see [illegible] form)

Plan of Care and Admission Orders Telephone Orders Received
By [signature], MD
Date 4/26 Time 1:50 p

Plan of Care and Admission Orders
Physician's Signature [signature]
Date 4-27 Time

Plan of Care and Admission Orders
Orders Noted By [signature]
Date 04-26-00 Time

FAX ORIGINAL TO PHARMACY SEND CARBON IN TOTE PAGE 2 OF 2

FORM 133PC/AD Reorder From: MED-PASS 800-438-8884 XFM 102298

Figure 2b: Admission orders, page 2 of 2 – activities to be performed by nursing staff.

What concerns the nursing home administrators, though, is not a pleasant moment for the patient but rather protecting their ability to receive an uninterrupted stream of reimbursement from Medicare.

Seven lines down on the second page's right side, you will find the heading "catheter" and below that the notation "IFC, FR18 Q month." This indicates that the patient has been given an in-dwelling Foley catheter, size French 18 (the diameter of a pencil) that will be changed only once a month. (A urinary catheter, which is not always necessary from the patient's perspective, is a long rubber tube that is inserted into the bladder to drain urine into a bag.) This tells you that the home views this patient as likely to be a long-term resident, and that the goal is not to change diapers or take out the catheter – or even review the situation – if at all possible. Urinary catheters are often medically unnecessary and in fact can create problems, such as urinary tract infections. The misuse of urinary catheters, which are often more helpful to the staff than they are to the patient, is a violation that state surveyors frequently cite.

Make Your Desires Known

To avoid situations that might cause your loved one discomfort, it is important to make your desires known. On the day the patient is admitted, visualize what you want done for him or her. If what you or the patient desire is not in the physician's orders, it is unlikely it will ever be performed. For example, your mother might really enjoy a glass of wine each day or a bowl of ice cream at bedtime. If her health permits, she should have it. Make her choices known and insist they be honored unless there is good reason for them not to be.

Family members are often reluctant to suggest treatment to a physician. You're obviously not going to tell the doctor what drug to use, but you can ask that certain situations be addressed. You don't want Mom to be in pain, for instance, so you might inquire what the doctor has ordered to help her sleep comfortably at night. More important, you might ask what plan has been put into place to ensure she receives pain medication. If the doctor prescribes Tylenol "as needed" for pain every four hours, this puts the responsibility for requesting the medication on the patient.

This is not where you want the responsibility to lie. Ask what active steps will be taken to evaluate Mom's pain every four hours. Better yet, insist that while your mother is awake a staff member perform a pain evaluation every four hours in addition to offering her the medication. Or, you might just want her to receive the medication every night before bedtime unless there is some reason not to do so.

Another situation you might address would be that urinary catheter. What has the doctor ordered to eliminate the pain of the insertion and removal of the device? Has the physician prescribed any medication that will reduce the constant urge to urinate when the catheter is in place? Most of the time nothing will be given unless you make a request. The routine procedure for placement and replacement of in-dwelling catheters involves washing the area to maintain sterility and using K-Y jelly or a similar substance for lubrication. Unfortunately, this bare-bones approach can cause great discomfort to the patient.

A more humane method would be to use lidocaine jelly, which is a local anesthetic, instead of the K-Y. Even better would be for the patient to be pre-medicated with pain-reducing drugs in addition to using the lidocaine jelly. You can be sure that this is what most doctors would ask for if they found themselves in this situation. Should the doctor respond, "It's not so bad, I wouldn't use lidocaine even for a family member of mine," tell him that, regardless, you want your mom to be treated better. You'll be happy to know that federal law now requires providers to develop, evaluate, and revise a patient's treatment plan with regard to pain.

Medicare pays the physician for only one nursing home visit a month for routine care, so make it count. Have a written list of questions and requests ready.

Physician's Orders

We'll use the same method we used above to review physician's orders (Figure 3). Here again, the example is well organized, legible, for the correct patient, and involves providers and activities of all types. Did you notice the dates – charting for 6/01/00 through 6/30/00 – near the bottom? The typed orders are automatic physician's orders that will continue each month unless specifically discontinued. You can see why you want to have your orders noted by the physician. Once orders are in place, they remain so until the doctor cancels them.

With this style of orders, the proper way to alter treatment is not to say "increase Tylenol from two tablets every six hours to two tablets every four hours" but rather: 1) Discontinue Tylenol two tablets every six hours; and 2) Start Tylenol two tablets every four hours. The date and time would be recorded next to these orders. The next month the new orders would be inserted, all nicely typed out.

An indication of this can be seen in the left column near the bottom, "Orders Brought Forward 5/27/00." The order for Megace, an appetite enhancer, was transferred from the previous record to a new one. The family could have suggested that an order be written that the

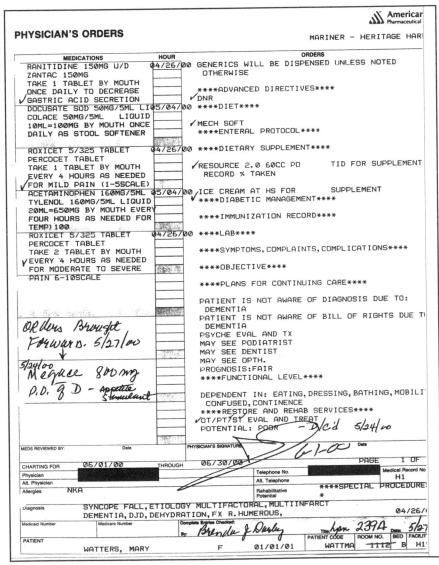

Figure 3: Physician's orders – medication and treatment regimens.

Required Insulin Checks Not Documented

a. The resident had a physician's order dated 10/15/00 for sliding scale insulin based on the results of accuchecks [monitoring of a diabetic's glucose level] to be done before meals, at bedtime and at 1:00 a.m.

b. The November 2000 MARS had a total of 37 skips where accuchecks were not documented and 18 skips where insulin administration was not documented.

— State survey, Warren, Arkansas, December 7, 2000

patient's pain be evaluated and documented every four hours while awake. This shifts the responsibility for pain management from the patient to the nursing home staff. Patients suffering from dementia are not in a position to manage their pain properly.

The observant among you will notice that the name of the home is listed below the name of the pharmaceutical supplier in the top right corner of the form. You have likely received notes from your doctor written on stationery supplied by a drug company. Not only is American Pharmaceutical on the stationery, but the company also is the default supplier of all pharmaceuticals for this home. And here is the kicker: At the time the order was written, American Pharmaceutical was a subsidiary of Mariner Health Group, the home's parent corporation.

Interim Order Forms

Once again, evaluate the interim order form (Figure 4) as a whole before looking at the specifics. The document is filled in completely by hand, and includes the correct patient and facility name. The entry dates are in proper sequence and the notations for each day are the same. "NNO" – shorthand for "no new orders" – appears over and over. The rest of the shorthand stands for "24-hour chart check." All this is followed on each line by a signature with title (LPN, or licensed practical nurse).

This sheet could have new orders written to alleviate suffering and discomfort, but evidently the patient had no problems that required an entry from at least June 21 through July 1. This patient would appear to be on remote control, and the purpose of the NNO notations is to protect the nurses. No matter what happens, the nurses will answer, "It didn't happen on my shift" and "The doctor didn't order anything for that."

Did you notice the pharmacy name change in the upper right-hand corner? American Pharmaceutical is no longer doing the work. Now it's NeighborCare. As with the original assignment of a pharmaceutical provider, this change was made without explanation.

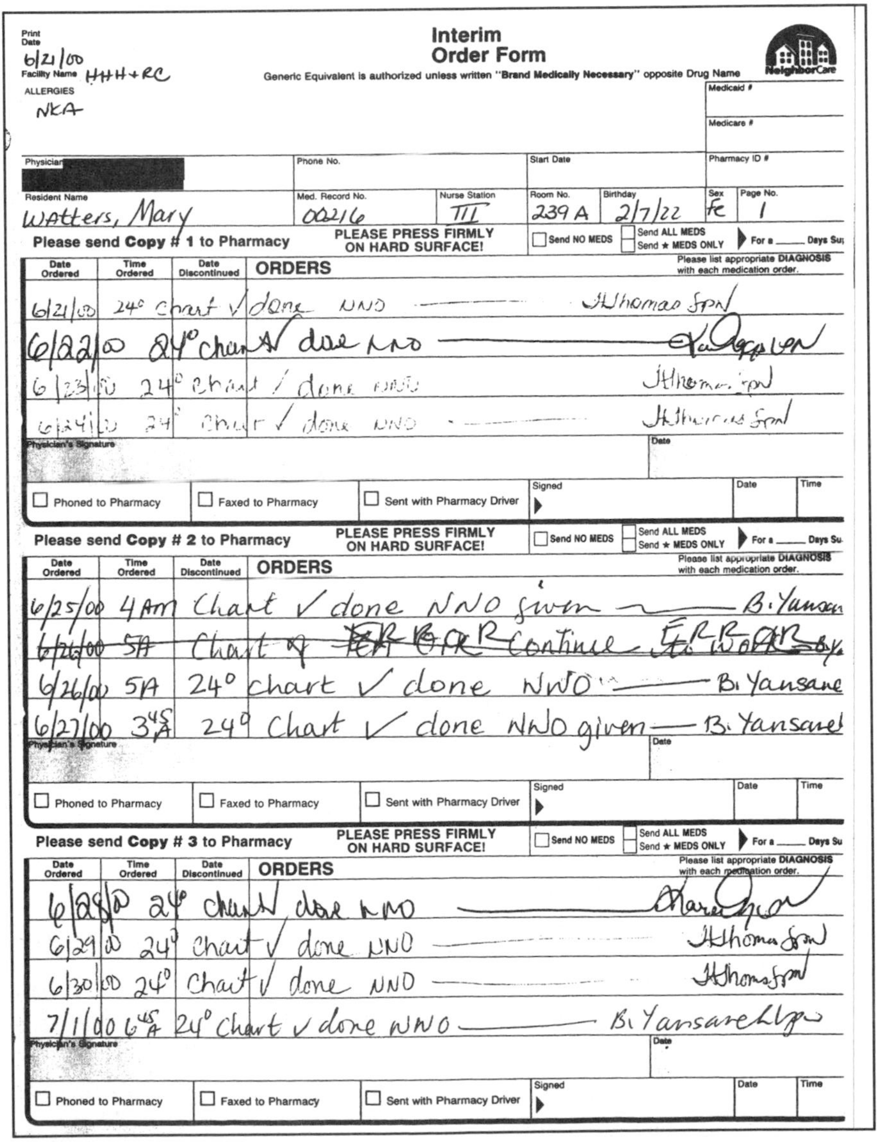

Figure 4: *Interim orders, staff notes, and additional providers' orders.*

5
PHYSICIAN/PROGRESS NOTES

Attending physicians know what goes on in nursing homes, but self-interest sometimes prevents them from doing anything about problems they witness. The best way to absolve themselves of responsibility is through careful documentation in their portion of the medical record, known as physician notes – also called progress notes, though "progress" is a misnomer if you are under the impression that your loved one is receiving prescribed treatments and moving along toward recovery. Rather than follow the true scientific method and record detailed notes, which would allow for the replication of an experiment, the goal here is to limit the physician's liability while at the same time producing sufficient documentation to justify reimbursement.

This is a tough balancing act, but it's one that is performed thousands of times a day.

The SOAP Format

The ideal progress note will be broken into four sections, in what is known as the SOAP format:

- Symptoms
- Objective findings
- Assessment
- Plan

Symptoms are generally observations made by the patient. You should also be recording your own list of symptoms that the patient talks about, as well as your objectives, assessments, and plans. "Mom complains of a wet diaper every day," is a symptom. When you lift the covers and see a urine-and-feces-contaminated bedsore and smell the acrid odor from her rotting flesh, that is an objective finding.

Though a patient may complain of symptoms of pain and physical discomfort, rarely if ever will you see any documentation of this when

Physician Fails to Sign and Date Orders and Notes

The physician must review the resident's total program of care, including medications and treatments, at each visit [and] write, sign, and date progress notes at each visit; and sign and date all orders.

This requirement is not met as evidenced by:

Based on record review and interview with licensed staff, the facility failed to obtain a dated physician signature for orders for two residents (#1 and #6). Findings:

Resident #1's current physician's orders for medications, treatments and care have not been signed since 10/12/00. The 10/12/00 physician's orders indicated they were for 60 days only. This finding was verified by licensed staff.

Resident #6's current order for medications, treatments and care [has] not been signed since 7/25/00. The 7/25/00 physician's orders indicated they were for 60 days only. This finding was verified by licensed staff.

– State survey, Howland, Maine, January 5, 2001

it involves the nursing staff, the facility, or the physical environment. Should a physician document anything negative concerning the nursing staff, its members would make life miserable by contacting her or him at all hours of the day and night to report on the patient.

Objective findings include the results of a physical examination and lab data. The note could include observations about breathing; heart and bowel sounds; the presence, size, and location of bruises, skin tears, and bedsores; and a host of other easily monitored conditions. But it probably won't. Just as you will have difficulty in finding all the pieces of the medical record, so does your doctor, who often has one additional impediment. Many physicians try to examine patients from the doorway. It's quicker – imagine the time saved by not having to wash hands between patients. Remember, if your loved one is on Medicaid, the doctor may not be making enough on this visit to order a large pizza with two toppings.

Your objective findings, on the other hand, might include "2 x 3-inch red area under diaper. See photo 10/23/2001, 5 p.m." If your observations don't match the physician's, or if things are left out, document your findings in a short note and send it to the attending physician,

Drugs Are Administered Without an Assessment

Based upon record review on 03/08/01 for sample resident #7, it was determined that the facility had initiated anti-psychotic drug therapy on 11/30/00 for the resident, without a prior assessment identifying an appropriate indication for therapy or alternative approaches to identify other possible causes for the behavioral symptoms the resident was experiencing . . . .

There was no documentation on that date by the physician in the resident's record indicating why the initiation of anti-psychotic therapy on 11/30/00 was clinically appropriate. No facility assessment was found in the record prior to that date to indicate the nature of the delusions, and there was no assessment found to indicate that the resident had functionally declined at that time.

– State survey, Midwest City, Oklahoma, March 1, 2001

the medical director, the nursing director, and the home's administrator. If you have power of attorney, you also have the right under the Health Insurance Portability and Accountability Act of 1996 (HIPAA) to request that amendments be made to the medical records. You should check with the nursing facility to obtain its written policy regarding its procedures for allowing these amendments to the records.

The physician's **assessment** should include a diagnosis based on the patient's symptoms and the objective findings and should include observations about the effectiveness of previous treatments. If you don't see a physician's assessment in the notes, ask about it, document what you are told, and then confirm the answer in writing to the director of nursing, the administrator, and the medical director to avoid any misunderstandings.

You should also be formulating your own assessment – such as "poor nursing care: bedsores" – and letting the nursing home administration and staff know. If your assessment is incorrect, you can be sure they will inform you. For sample letters to the administrator and the medical director see this book's Appendices, where you will also find tips on photographing your findings.

Treatment **plans** are the written intentions of the physician regarding future care. Under ideal circumstances the physician should list under the plans portion of the form the actions required of the staff and the medication and other orders that will result in amelioration of the problems listed in the assessment. Some plans may be very brief such as "continue to follow," "check weight once per week and order tests A, B, and C," "get patient out of bed twice per day," or "clean bedsores each shift and chart progress." The purpose of the plan is to state the problems and the method for treating them. The solution should include not only the specific active treatments but also some indication as to how progress will be monitored. (The part about monitoring progress might not always be spelled out in detail.)

Shifting Responsibility

Treatment plans are one area in which the doctor sometimes tries to shift responsibility to the family or patient. For example, the physician may write "loss of weight, bedsores secondary to decreased caloric intake. Family aware no hope for improvement without tube feedings. Family/patient refuses." What the physician has not addressed is the cause of the decreased caloric intake. The physician should ideally make an assessment and develop a treatment plan that correctly identifies the patient's limitations and available nursing home resources.

For example, if the patient is noted to have difficulty swallowing, an order for an evaluation by a speech pathologist is in order. If the patient has no teeth, a liquid or pureed diet might be appropriate, especially if the facility is known for serving food as tough as shoe leather. There are a host of remedies that can be pursued prior to initiating artificial tube feedings. However, the reason that may not have occurred is that tube feedings are doubly advantageous to the facility: they generate more reimbursement income and simultaneously decrease staff time per resident.

From a labor perspective, tube feeding comes down to the length of time it takes to hang a bottle of dinner on an IV pole compared with having a nursing assistant hand-feed pureed meals to a patient. A physician may suggest tube feeding because his experience with staff members hand-feeding patients often results in hungry patients and significant weight loss. The doctor knows this, or should know, but he is often disinclined to mention it to the family.

How to Review Progress Notes

May 6, 2000

Take a general look at the first progress note (Figure 5) of four we'll review. The writing is neat, aligned, and apparently organized, and the note is dated and signed.

The careful among you will notice, though, that two key items are missing: the patient's name and, more significantly, any writing on much of the page. That's an awful lot of empty space just waiting for an inappropriate entry at a later time. If the doctor who wrote the next note had wanted to start on a fresh page, there should have been a line

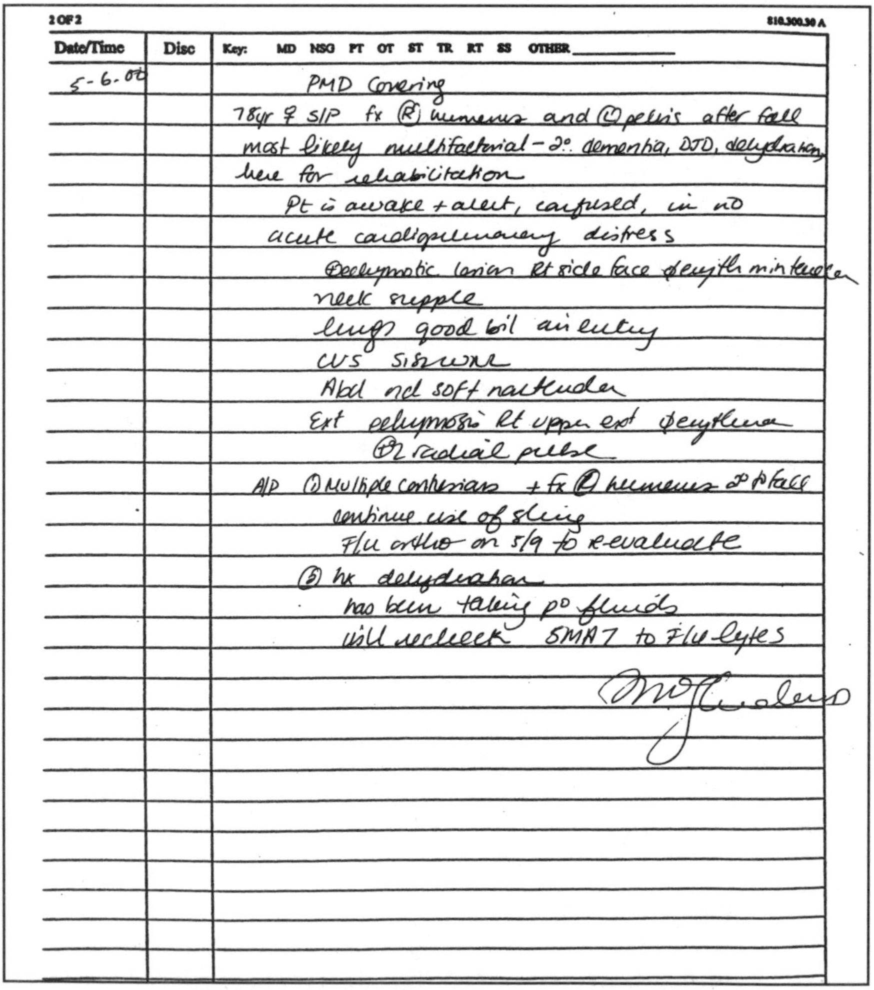
2 OF 2 810.300.30 A

Date/Time	Disc	Key: MD NSG PT OT ST TR RT SS OTHER ____
5-6-00		PMD Covering
		78yr ♀ S/P fx (R) humerus and (L) pelvis after fall
		most likely multifactorial – 2°. dementia, DJD, dehydration,
		here for rehabilitation
		Pt is awake + alert, confused, in no
		acute cardiopulmonary distress
		Ecchymotic lesion Rt side face with min tender
		neck supple
		lungs good b/l air entry
		CVS S1S2 WNL
		Abd nd soft nontender
		Ext ecchymosis Rt upper ext erythema
		(+)2 radial pulse
		A/P (1) Multiple contusions + fx (R) humerus 2° to fall
		continue use of sling
		F/u ortho on 5/9 to re-evaluate
		(3) hx dehydration
		has been taking po fluids
		will recheck SMA7 to F/u lytes
		[illegible signature]

Figure 5: Physician/progress note, 5/6/2000.

crossing out the rest of the first page. If another note goes in here out of sequence, whether done on purpose or not, this is wrong. If staff members make entries at a later time to cover their tracks, the veracity of the entire chart is presumed to be in doubt.

(To ensure against backdated entries and other shenanigans, you should periodically request a copy of the medical record. Every month or two, ask for a complete copy of the record. You'll likely be asked why you want to do this. Say you're making sure you haven't missed a page. At the time of discharge, get a copy of the entire chart and start to compare.)

See how much of the progress note you can understand on your own. Below is the translation:

Line No. Description

1. 5/6/2000 Primary medical doctor (PMD) covering ("Covering" means that another doctor is seeing the patient in place of the primary doctor, in this particular case on a Saturday.)
2. 78-year-old female with a fracture of the right humerus and left pelvis after a fall
3. Most likely multifactorial (due to more than one cause) secondary to dementia, degenerative joint disease, dehydration
4. Here for rehabilitation
5. Patient (Pt) is awake and alert, confused, in no
6. acute cardiopulmonary distress (heart and lungs seem okay).
7. Presence of ecchymotic lesion right side of face without erythema (bruise, not inflamed or infected)
8. Neck is supple (no stiffness)
9. Lungs good bilateral air entry (able to breathe with no air flow problems)
10. CVS S1S2WNL (Cardiovascular within normal limits; heart is normal)
11. Abdomen normal soft and nontender (belly doesn't hurt to touch, no swelling)
12. Extremities: ecchymoses right upper extremity without erythema (bruise right upper arm no redness)

Missing Label Results in a Medication Error

In describing Figure 5 we noted that the patient's name was omitted from the chart. The state survey report below illustrates the consequences of improper or missing labels, in this case of a room:

After the...medications were prepared, they were taken to the resident in the unlabeled resident room. The resident in this room received the 2 oral medications and swallowed them. When the medication nurse told the resident that there were eye drops that needed to be put in her eye, the resident asked, "Why do I need eye drops? What are they (eye drops) for?" The medication nurse stated, "The doctor ordered them. They're for your glaucoma." The resident then stated, "Well, I don't know. Do they go in both eyes?" The resident was informed they only went into her left eye. The eye drops were placed in the resident's left eye by the medication nurse.

The review of the above medication pass revealed that the medication nurse had passed 6 medications in error to the resident in the unlabeled room (resident 28). The medications that were given to resident 28 were the medications ordered for resident 29. The medication nurse did not report these medication errors.

– State survey, Salt Lake City, Utah, December 12, 2000

13. Radial pulse noted (patient has pulse in the radial artery by wrist each arm: no blockage)
14. Assessment/Plan (A/P) (1) Multiple contusions with fracture of right humerus secondary to fall
15. Continue to use sling
16. Follow up (F/U) appointment with orthopedic surgeon on May 9 to reevaluate
17. History of dehydration
18. Has been taking fluids by mouth
19. Will recheck lab work (sma7) to follow up on electrolytes
20. (Doctor's signature)

By most criteria, this is an excellent note. The only thing of importance that is missing is whether or not the patient had any complaints. From the appearance of the note, it is clear that this physician not only

Pressure Sore Worsens When Orders Aren't Followed

At 6:35 a.m. on 06/07/00 resident was observed in bed on right side with foam block support encircling right ankle....Bloody drainage was observed on ankle, foam support and bed linens. Wound was not covered with dressing.

...Observation by licensed nurse revealed wound Stage III, sizing approximately 2 cm. Depth was not determined due to bloody appearance of wound.

Pressure sore report showed no documentation regarding ankle since 04/23/00 when pressure sore developed. At that time ankle was Stage II, 1.2 cm x 0.7 cm with 0.1 cm depth without drainage. . . .

Physician progress notes from 04/23/00 indicated treatment for pressure sore was hydrogel and bandaid daily until healed. On 05/11/00 physician stopped treatment to ankle and ordered right foot to be in foam block left open to air. Progress notes from physician indicated resident had poor tissues but no peripheral vascular disease and pressure sore was from pressure. Interview with charge nurse on 06/07/00 at 10:00 a.m. revealed that each Tuesday all pressure sores were to be looked at and documented on the pressure ulcer report sheet. There was no wound documentation done for Tuesday, 06/06/00.

– State survey, Elwood, Nebraska, June 14, 2000

examined the patient but also reviewed the chart. There is no way from the patient he would have known about the dehydration, fractures, and circumstances of her admission.

Looking at the physical portion of the exam, you can see he started at the head and worked down. It's not clear whether he examined the patient's feet or the skin on the coccyx, or tailbone, but let's give him the benefit of the doubt. The physician's assessment and plan, though perhaps not complete, addressed the major concerns he noticed by looking at both the patient and the chart.

It is evident that the note was intended to provide information for the patient's usual primary medical doctor, and that it was meant to be read and understood.

May 24, 2000

Now let's look at a note (Figure 6) written by the patient's personal physician (coincidentally, the medical director of the facility) about 18 days later.

Once again, look at the note generally. What is your impression? A good guess would be that the doctor was in a hurry and that this was one of many patients he was seeing that day. The name isn't filled out, there is no full date, and the time isn't noted. Without some experience, about the only thing you can make out is that something

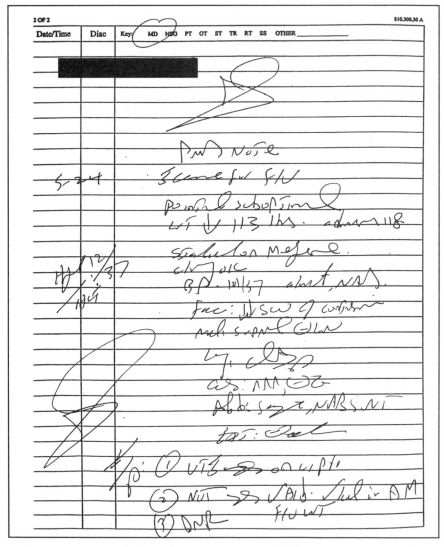

Figure 6: Physician/progress note, 5/24/2000.

decreased to 113 and the DNR (Do Not Resuscitate) at the end of the note. This note serves to document a visit for the purpose of billing and perhaps a little bit more.

The rough translation of the note is as follows:

Line No.   *Description*

1. (Doctor's signature)
2. PMD note
3. 5/24 (/2000) Without complaints came for follow up
4. PO intake (oral intake) suboptimal
5. Weight has decreased to 113 pounds from the admission weight of 118 pounds
6. Currently on Megace (a drug to increase appetite)
7. Not legible (To the left: Hgb/Hct: 12/37– hemoglobin/hematocrit are low and indicate anemia)
8. (Blood pressure reading.) Alert, no acute distress
9. Face: decrease swelling of contusion (bruise)
10. Neck supple, no lymph nodes felt
11. Lungs clear to auscultation (heard patient breath with stethoscope)
12. Cardiovascular system: regular rhythm rate of heart, no gallops
13. Abdomen: soft normal active bowel sounds, nontender
14. Extremities: no edema
    (1) Urinary tract infection (UTI); on Cipro
    (2) (Illegible) check (illegible) in a.m.
    (3) Do Not Resuscitate (DNR) "follow up weight"

The notes in the physical examination are almost pro forma. This does not mean the doctor didn't perform the examination, but the way the information is scribbled hardly inspires the confidence that the notes in the first example do. What do you think the odds are that the second doctor lifted the covers, examined the patient's back, buttocks, groin, fractured arm, and pelvis – not to mention checked out the vast array of data in the chart from the therapists, nurses, and other staff members? The decrease in weight is noted, but the doctor didn't address the issue of diet.

June 20, 2000

Perhaps May 24 was just a bad day, so let's look at the note written 27 days later (Figure 7). The patient's weight is now 104 pounds, and her family doesn't want her tube fed. The physical examination is nearly identical in form and content to the previous one. So what was the purpose of this note? To document that the family was aware of the weight loss, had refused tube feedings, and that the doctor had consulted the dietician – which is to say shifted all responsibility from him.

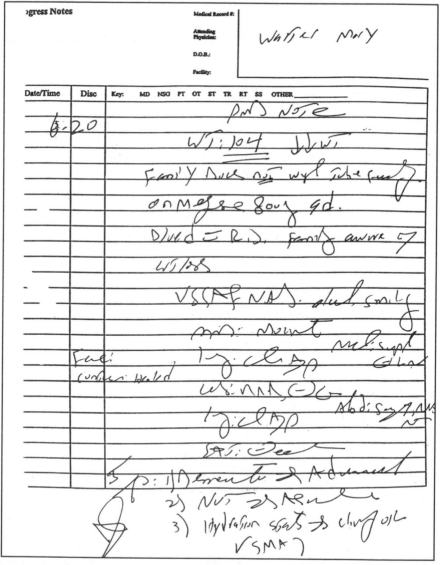

Figure 7: Physician/progress note, 6/20/2000.

Here is the translation:

Line No.   *Description*

1.   PMD note
2.   June 20, 2000
3.   Weight: 104 pounds; decrease in weight
4.   Family does not want tube feedings
5.   On Megace, 800mg per day
6.   Discussed with registered dietician that family is aware of
7.   weight loss
8.   Vital signs stable, afebrile (no fever), no acute distress, alert and smiling
9.   (Illegible)
10. Neck supple (no stiffness), no lymph nodes (no bumps in neck)
11. Lungs clear to auscultation and percussion (lungs appear normal by listening and tapping on chest)
12. Facial contusions (bruises) healed
13. Exam of heart shows regular rhythm and rate with no gallop
14. Abdomen soft, normal active bowel sounds, nontender
15. Lungs clear to auscultation and percussion (the doctor has twice written the same thing – talk about being pro forma)
16. Extremities without edema (no swelling)
17. Assessment and plan
     (1) Dementia, advanced
     (2) (Illegible)
     (3) Hydration (illegible) OK
     (4) Check sma7 (a series of lab tests)
18. (Doctor's signature)

The above type of documentation is not only proper: it is required. What makes it unacceptable is the doctor's lack of attention to nearly everything else going on with the patient.

July 24, 2000

Still need convincing? Look at the next example (Figure 8), from July 24. The patient's weight is now 94.7 pounds, and the physical exam is nearly identical to the previous ones. There's also the obligatory note about "no tube feeding per family." The assessment and plan: weight loss, on Megace, prognosis poor, advanced dementia.

Here's the translation:

Line No.   *Description*

1.   PMD note
2.   7/24/2000; Weight 94.7 pounds (down 7-10 pounds)
3.   No tube feeding per family.
4.   RD (registered dietician) note checked
5.   Vital signs stable, afebrile, no acute distress
6.   Patient alert, confused
7.   Neck supple
8.   Lungs clear to auscultation and percussion –
      to left: TSH OK follow up 6 weeks (TSH is thyroid
      stimulating hormone)
9.   Cardiac regular rhythm and rate no gallops (normal)
10.   Abdomen: soft normal active bowel sounds, nontender
11.   Extremities: no edema (no swelling in ankles, hands, etc.)
12.   Assessment/Plan:
      (1) Weight loss, patient on Megace
          Prognosis poor
      (2) Advanced dementia

13.   (Doctor's signature)

Can you identify what is missing in this note? The first part should address the symptoms and history as obtained from the patient and notes from other providers of care. There should be a lot more to discuss than the decrease in weight, but the record contains nothing about the fractures, the condition of the skin, the presence of contractures (shortening of tendons in the arms and legs, causing the patient to lapse into the fetal position; this occurs when no physical therapy is provided), the patient's fluid or caloric intake, or any review of the notes from the dietician, nurse, physical therapist, or the speech therapist.

Back to our previous question. What was the purpose of this entry? It certainly was not to convey information to other providers or detail a plan that would address the needs of this patient. Rather, it was to transfer responsibility for the 19.7 percent drop in body weight from the facility to the patient and family.

Ask for a Translation

The four notes we have reviewed cover a period of 79 days. As it happens, these were the only notes from the private physician during that time frame. He visited about every 30 days – what most states require, and what Medicare will reimburse. You may have thought we were being harsh before, but these notes show what goals are being fulfilled: get the money and shift the blame. Next patient, please.

When you review a progress note, don't be afraid to ask for a translation. Remember your goals and see if the items on your list have been addressed. Open-ended questions are fine. For example, "I see that the nurses are looking at ways to prevent or treat my mother's bedsores. Doctor, what have you found, and what are your suggestions?"

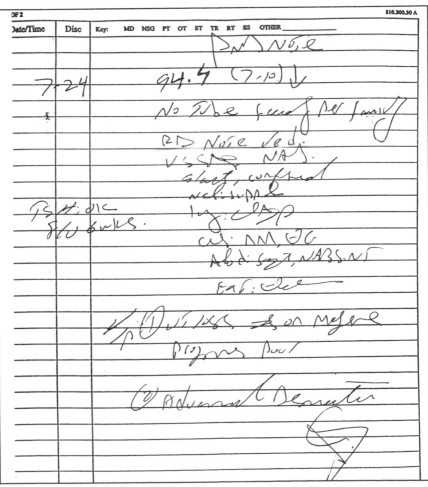

Figure 8: Physician/progress note, 7/24/2000.

6
NURSING NOTES

Nurses document everything. They sign off on the physician's orders, transcribe the orders to their own forms, note that they have followed the orders, record every bowel movement the patient makes and the intake of food or drink, and account for just about every other activity that occurs. Nurses also document that the physician was notified of every conceivable finding, thus relieving themselves and the facility of any culpability should things go awry. They have their own set of records, which in general are much better than those of the physicians, though you need to know how to detect falsification.

The important ingredients for a complete set of nursing notes, described below and with examples, include the following: contemporaneous notes, the MDS (Minimum Data Set), the RAP (Resident Assessment Protocol), care plans, a weight chart, a skin chart, and MARS (Medication Administration Record System) and TARS (Treatment Administration Record System) reports.

Contemporaneous Notes
The contemporaneous notes are those made from day to day. These notes would include observations about the smell of the urine, the look of a bedsore, and what findings the physician was made aware of. Figure 9 represents a typical set of such notes.

As with the physician notes, first review the page as a whole. It is concise, with almost no space between entries. It is dated, but there is no patient name.

Now, let's look at the details, the most significant of which is that there are no entries for 45 days, from June 21 until August 5. What with the patient losing weight and suffering from contractures, bedsores, and other side effects of living in a nursing home, you would think there would be nursing notes covering this period. There should have been, and in fact this is a significant clue that something has gone very wrong.

When you examine the nursing notes, first look at the dates. Are there any large gaps between entries? With this set of records, the next question to ask is why the notes start up again on August 5. It appears as though the patient's daughter was notified of a skin tear on the right arm, and that the attending physician was notified by pager regarding treatment orders. The addendum to the August 5 entry discusses how the area was cleaned and dressed.

In this particular instance, what the medical record doesn't include is that a defective chair with sharp edges caused the skin tears and that when the family found the arm bandaged and inquired about the

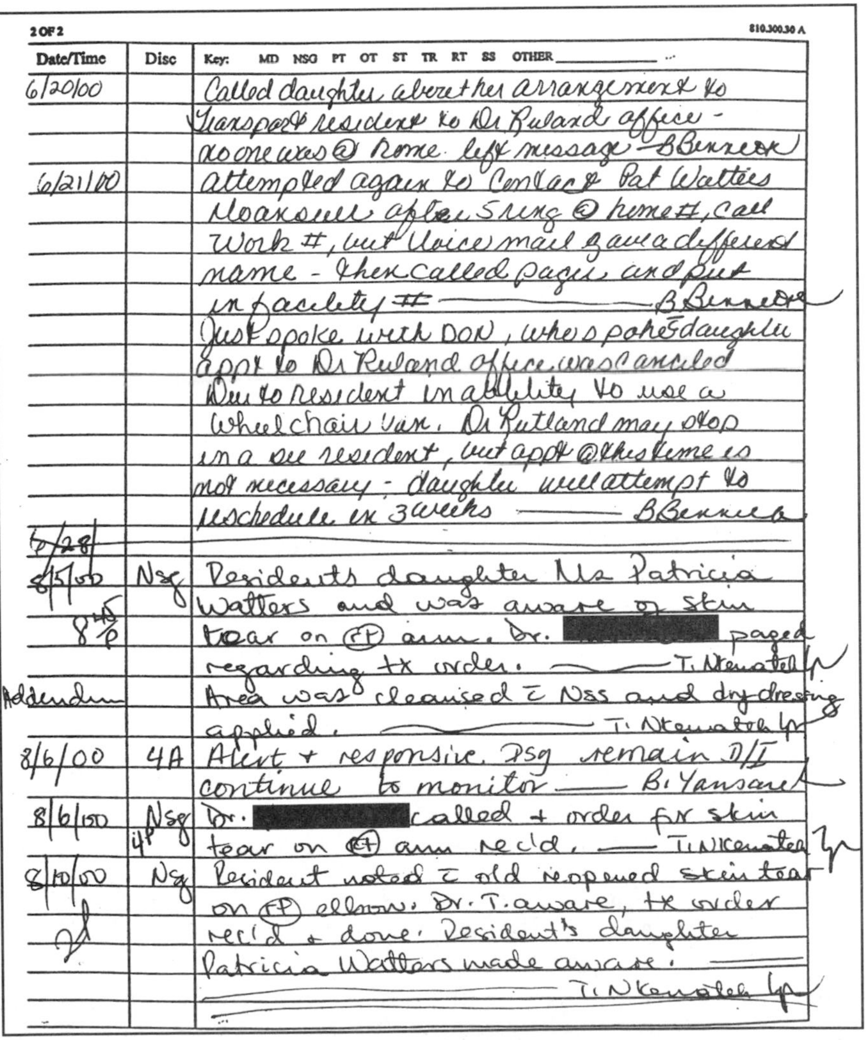

2 OF 2 810.300.30 A

Date/Time	Disc	Key: MD NSG PT OT ST TR RT SS OTHER ______
6/20/00		Called daughter about her arrangement to transport resident to Dr Ruland office - no one was @ home. left message - B Bennett
6/21/00		attempted again to contact Pat Watters Noansell after 5 ring @ home #, call Work #, but voice mail gave a different name - then called pager and put in facility # ——— B Bennett
		Just spoke with DON, who spoke daughter appt to Dr Ruland office was cancelled due to resident inability to use a wheelchair van. Dr Rutland may stop in a see resident, but appt @ this time is not necessary - daughter will attempt to reschedule in 3 weeks ——— B Bennett
~~6/28~~		
8/5/00 8:45p	Nsg	Residents daughter Ms Patricia Watters and was aware of skin tear on (Rt) arm. Dr. [redacted] paged regarding tx order. ——— T. Nkemateh lpn
Addendum		Area was cleansed c NSS and dry dressing applied. ——— T. Nkemateh lpn
8/6/00	4A	Alert + responsive. Dsg remain D/I continue to monitor ——— B. Yansane
8/6/00 4p	Nsg	Dr. [redacted] called + order for skin tear on (Rt) arm rec'd. ——— T. Nkemateh lpn
8/10/00 2d	Nsg	Resident noted c old reopened skin tear on (Rt) elbow. Dr. T. aware, tx order rec'd + done. Resident's daughter Patricia Watters made aware. ——— T. Nkemateh lpn

Figure 9: *Nursing notes from 6/20/2000 to 8/10/2000.*

No Plan to Prevent Recurrence of Bruises

Based on record review and staff interview, the facility failed to assess bruises of unknown origin...documentation in the medical record noted a 4 x 2 cm purple bruise on the resident's right arm. There was no additional documentation or assessment in the record of the bruise and how it may have occurred. Thus there was no plan to prevent recurrence.

— State survey, Yakima, Washington, October 11, 2000

mishap they were told, "It didn't happen on my shift, I don't know anything about it." What the nurses have done is buff the chart, the purpose of which is to provide sufficient documentation to support a selective version of events. It's like polishing a car: just keep rubbing until it looks better. Always read nursing notes with this in mind. If something has happened and it is not recorded, you need to insist on the documentation.

Minimum Data Set

Nurses' lives revolve around "process," a term used to describe their activities as they perform a series of tasks related to compiling the Minimum Data Set, or MDS for short. Figure 10 is a page from an MDS form, for which entries are required on admission, quarterly, with a significant change in condition, annually, or to correct previous errors. If submitted for Medicare services, data must be collected on days 5, 14, 30, 60, and 90. Special rules also apply for patients who are admitted to a hospital or are returning from a hospital stay. This data, which the state and the federal Center for Medicare & Medicaid Services (CMS) collect as part of the certification process, is a basic instrument for documenting and performing a proper assessment of a nursing home patient.

Below is a description, excerpted from documents produced by the CMS, of the tasks involved in compiling an MDS:

> *Assessment:* taking stock of all observations, information and knowledge about a resident; understanding the resident's limitations and strengths; finding out who the resident is. In essence, the MDS is a tool for assessment.

Decision-Making: Determining the severity, functional impact, and scope of a resident's problems; understanding the causes and relationships between a resident's problems; discovering the "whats" and "whys" of resident problems.

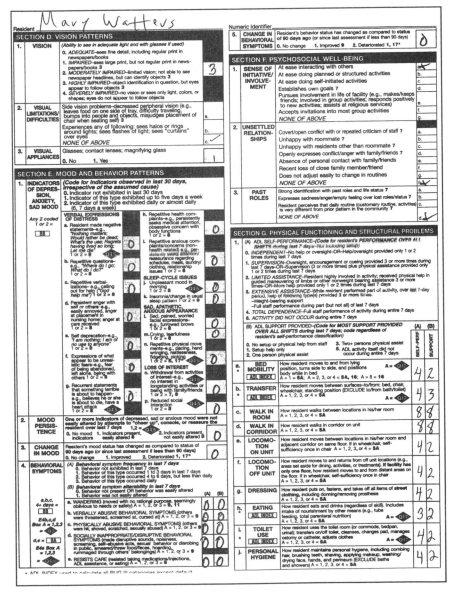

Figure 10: MDS–Minimum Data Set, selected sections.

Resident Assessment Protocol

The RAP, or Resident Assessment Protocol, is what guides the decision-making process. As you can see from Figure 11, a section of a Resident Assessment Protocol Summary, nurses check off items they have observed while compiling the MDS. You will notice that in several cases on the summary, RAP has been "triggered," meaning that the nurses must then follow RAP guidelines to determine other areas that might need assessment.

Required for Comprehensive Assessments
SECTION V. RESIDENT ASSESSMENT PROTOCOL SUMMARY   Numeric Identifier___

Resident's Name: _Mary Watters_   Medical Record No.: _00216_

1. Check if RAP is triggered.
2. For each triggered RAP, use the RAP guidelines to identify areas needing further assessment. Document relevant assessment information regarding the resident's status.
   - Describe:
     –Nature of the condition (may include presence or lack of objective data and subjective complaints).
     –Complications and risk factors that affect your decision to proceed to care planning.
     –Factors that must be considered in developing individualized care plan interventions.
     –Need for referrals/further evaluation by appropriate health professionals.
   - Documentation should support your decision–making regarding whether to proceed with a care plan for a triggered RAP and the type(s) of care plan interventions that are appropriate for a particular resident.
   - Documentation may appear anywhere in the clinical record (e.g., progress notes, consults, flowsheets, etc.).
3. Indicate under the <u>Location of RAP Assessment Documentation</u> column where information related to the RAP assessment can be found.
4. For each triggered RAP, indicate whether a new care plan, care plan revision, or continuation of current care plan is necessary to address the problem(s) identified in your assessment. The Care Planning Decision column must be completed within 7 days of completing the RAI (MDS and RAPs).

A. RAP Problem Area	(a) Check if Triggered	Location and Date of RAP Assessment Documentation	(b) Care Planning Decision–check if addressed in care plan
1. DELIRIUM	✓	See Rap	✓
2. COGNITIVE LOSS	✓	See Rap	
3. VISUAL FUNCTION	✓	See Rap	✓
4. COMMUNICATION	✓	See Rap	✓
5. ADL FUNCTIONAL/ REHABILITATION POTENTIAL	✓	See Rap	✓
6. URINARY INCONTINENCE AND INDWELLING CATHETER	✓	See Rap	
7. PSYCHOSOCIAL WELL-BEING			
8. MOOD STATE			
9. BEHAVIORAL SYMPTOMS			
10. ACTIVITIES			
11. FALLS	✓	See Rap	✓
12. NUTRITIONAL STATUS	✓	See Rap	✓
13. FEEDING TUBES			
14. DEHYDRATION/FLUID MAINTENANCE			
15. ORAL/DENTAL CARE			
16. PRESSURE ULCERS	✓	See Rap	✓
17. PSYCHOTROPIC DRUG USE			
18. PHYSICAL RESTRAINTS			

B. ___

1. Signature of RN Coordinator for RAP Assessment Process

3. Signature of Person Completing Care Planning Decision

Encode the MDS, edit, correct and lock no later than:

2. | 0 | 5 | – | 0 | 8 | – | 2 | 0 | 0 | 0 | → Completion date of Comprehensive Assessment (Assessment Lock date=VB2 + 7 days)
   Month   Day   Year

4. | 0 | 5 | – | 0 | 8 | – | 2 | 0 | 0 | 0 | → Completion date of Care Plan decision (Care Plan Lock date=VB4 + 7 days)
   Month   Day   Year

EDT Transmission error if all checkmarks and dates are not encoded (entered into and printed by a computer program)

®️ = Key items for computerized resident tracking – Key Field errors may be corrected by submitting a "Key Change Request" to the State.

Figure 11: Resident Assessment Protocol summary sheet.

All this data collection leads to the Care Plan, whose components, below, are also excerpted from CMS documents:

> *Care Planning:* Establishing a course of action that moves a resident toward a specific goal utilizing individual resident strengths and interdisciplinary expertise; crafting the "how" of resident care.

> *Implementation:* Putting that course of action... into motion by staff knowledgeable about the resident care goals and approaches: carrying out the "how" and "when" of resident care.

> *Evaluation:* Critically reviewing care plan goals, interventions and implementation in terms of achieved resident outcomes and assessing the need to modify the care plan...to adjust to changes in the resident's status, either improvement or decline.

The MDS, RAP, Care Plan and Implementation of the Care Plan form an interconnected system of how doctors and nurses collect and analyze patient data, as shown in Figure 12.

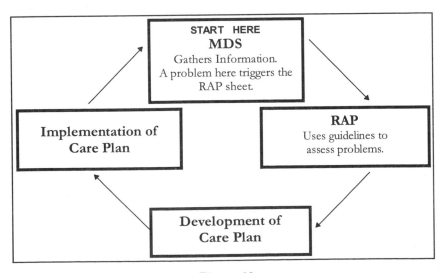

Figure 12

The RAP Module

One of the items checked on the Resident Assessment Protocol summary is nutritional status. The next step for the nurse is to answer questions relative to nutrition in the RAP Module titled Nutritional Status (Figure 13). The questions revolve around major areas that can affect nutrition, from medical, behavioral, and cognitive issues to ones related to function and communication.

NUTRITIONAL STATUS
MDS 2.0 RAP MODULE

INSTRUCTIONS: Identify the MDS 2.0 items that specifically triggered this RAP in the space provided and review the RAP Guidelines. Wor' section of this RAP Module at a time, check Yes, No, or Not Applicable (N/A) for each question asked. Use space available to expand, as app on any/all of your responses. At the end of each section, summarize and document your findings in the Summary of Findings section located on the reverse. Proceed to the next section. Once this has been done for all sections, review and analyze the *entire* Summary section and formulate your care planning decision.

What MDS 2.0 item(s) triggered this RAP? __K5__

MEDICAL FACTORS FOR CONSIDERATION   YES | NO | N/A

1. Does resident have a decreased or altered ability to taste or smell food? If Yes, specify by circling.
   Diarrhea *(H2c)*   Pneumonia *(I2e)*   Nutrient/Medication interactions
   Anemia *(I1oo)*   Fever *(J1h)*   Other: _____
   Cancer *(I1pp)*   Cancer therapy *(P1a)*

2. Has appetite decreased since administration of any of the following? If Yes, specify by circling.
   Antipsychotics *(O4a)*   Laxatives *(From record)*
   Cardiac Drugs *(From record)* Antacids *(From record)*
   Diuretics *(O4e)*   Other: _____

3. Does resident have constipation, intestinal obstruction or pain that would inhibit appetite? If Yes, specify: __Pain del__

4. Does resident have shortness of breath *(J1l)*, weakness, paleness of mucous membranes and nail beds and/or clubbing? If Yes, specify: _____

5. Based on the above review, are there medical condition(s) which are impacting the resident's nutritional status? Indicate Yes or No *and* specifically document your findings in the Summary of Findings section.

BEHAVIORAL FACTORS FOR CONSIDERATION   YES | N

1. Does resident use food to gain staff's attention? If Yes, specify: _____
2. Does resident behave in an anti-social or inappropriate manner (i.e, throws food) when dining with other residents? If Yes, specify: _____
3. Does resident have behavior problems that place him/her at risk for malnutrition? If Yes, specify by circling.
   Pacing *(E1n)*   Wandering *(E4a)*   Disruptive behavior *(E4d)*
4. Has resident withdrawn from activities of interest; being with family/friends; ADL self-performance? *(E1o)* If Yes, specify: _____
5. Based on the above review, are there behavioral factors which are impacting the resident's nutritional status? Indicate Yes or No *and* specifically document your findings in the Summary of Findings section.

COGNITIVE FACTORS FOR CONSIDERATION   YES | NO | N/A

1. Does resident have mental problems that place him/her at risk for malnutrition? If Yes, specify by circling.
   Mental retardation *(AB10)*   Alzheimer's *(I1q)*   Anxiety disorders *(I1dd)*
   Depression *(I1ee)*   Other dementia *(I1u)*   Other: _____
2. Does resident exhibit unwarranted fears (e.g., fear that food is poisoned; fear of swallowing)? *(E1; from record)* _____
3. Is resident able to understand the importance of eating? _____
4. Based on the above review, are there cognitive factor(s) which are impacting the resident's nutritional status? Indicate Yes or No *and* specifically document your findings in the Summary of Findings section.

Name—Last	First	Middle	Attending Physician	I.D. No.
Watters	Mary			00216

Form 1712NH © 1995 Briggs Corporation, Des Moines, IA 50306 (800) 247-2343 PRINTED IN U.S.A.   **Continued On Reverse**

Figure 13a: RAP module on nutritional status, page 1 of 2.

The questions in the RAP module direct the nurse in preparing the care plan. For example, under "Functional Factors for Consideration," the report notes that the patient has a reduced ability to feed herself and leaves 25 percent or more of her food uneaten. And the patient has suffered a loss of upper-extremity use. These factors indicate that at a minimum the patient would require assistance to eat. The family could then ask about staffing issues and whether arrangements had been made to be sure assistance was available at every meal.

NUTRITIONAL STATUS
MDS 2.0 RAP MODULE

FUNCTIONAL FACTORS FOR CONSIDERATION	YES	NO	N/A
Does resident have a reduced ability to feed self? *(G1h)* ___ If Yes: Does resident require assistance with feeding, adaptive equipment, specialized training? Specify: ___	✓		
2. Does resident leave 25% or more of food uneaten? *(K4c)* ___	✓		
3. Does resident have: a. An ostomy? *(H3I)* ___ b. Difficulty chewing? *(K1a)* ___ c. Poorly fitting dentures? ___ d. Difficulty swallowing? *(K1b)* ___	✓ ✓ ✓ ✓		
4. Is resident slow in feeding self? *(G8c)* ___		✓	
5. Has resident suffered the loss of upper-extremity use? *(G4a, b, c)* ___	✓		
6. Has resident had weight loss due to amputation? *(I1n)* ___		✓	
7. Based on the above review, are there functional factors which are impacting the resident's nutritional status? Indicate Yes or No *and* specifically document your findings in the Summary of Findings section.	✓		

COMMUNICATION FACTORS FOR CONSIDERATION	YES	NO	N/A
1. Does resident have difficulty making food/mealtime preferences/dislikes known? *(C3g, C4, C5, C6)*	✓		
2. Does resident's inability to communicate place him/her at risk for malnutrition? If Yes, specify: Comatose *(B1)* ⬭Decision making ability *(B4)*⬭ Aphasia *(I1r)* Other: ___	✓		
3. Based on the above review, are there communication factor(s) which are impacting the resident's nutritional status? Indicate Yes or No *and* specifically document your findings in the Summary of Findings section.	✓		

SUMMARY OF FINDINGS

NOTE: This documentation must support the criteria outlined in Instruction #2 on the Resident Assessment Protocol Summary (MDS 2.0, Section V.). In short, you must describe the nature of the problem; causes, complications and risk factors (including impact on health and well-being); and provide justification for proceeding or not proceeding to care planning.

See care plan #2. At risk for nutritional concerns. Proceed c̄
care plan.

CARE PLAN DECISION BASED ON SUMMARY ABOVE: ☒ Proceed with care planning ☐ Not proceed with care planning

Signature, Title & Dates of Staff Who Completed RAP

(signature) 5/8/0

Name—Last	First	Middle	Attending Physician	I.D. No.

Figure 13b: RAP module on nutritional status, page 2 of 2.

Interdisciplinary Care Plan

You can see the flow of information very easily from the Interdisciplinary Care Plan (Figure 14). The MDS is an instrument used to collect raw nursing information. This data is then used to identify patient problems, which are listed on the RAP sheet, and the RAP modules provide guidance to the nurses as to the factors involved in a given problem. The care plan specifies a particular problem, a goal, and approaches to solving the problem; lists the responsible parties;

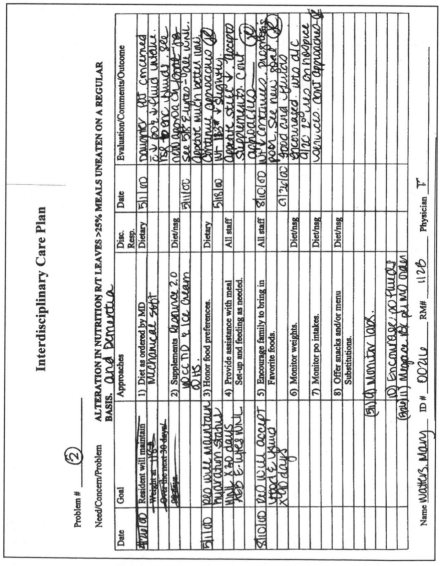

Figure 14: Interdisciplinary Care Plan.

Pain Continues Because No Plan Is in Place

Resident #9...sustained a fractured tibia on 8/4/00 and was being treated for same. The physician ordered pain medication (Darvocet-N 100 one tablet every 6 hours as needed). Review of the clinical record revealed that the nurses had documented many times that he/she was experiencing pain. The monthly summary dated 8/8/00 revealed, "Soft cast on left leg. Resident had been crying with pain every night since splint was applied. It is very disturbing to see something done that is hurting and making him/her cry. Is family aware?" Review of the comprehensive assessment, dated 8/9/00 revealed that the resident was experiencing moderate pain less than daily. This did not coincide with the nurse's notes. Review of the care plan for this resident, dated 08/09/00, revealed that there was no care plan in place to address pain management.

– State survey, Hobe Sound, Florida, November 8, 2000

and includes an evaluation, comments, and a desired outcome. This same process is followed for each problem identified. Care plans should be updated on a regular basis. As you can see, after mid-May no one looked again until August 10.

What to Ask to Review

So now you know what to ask for. Show me the:

- MDS
- RAP Sheet
- RAP Modules
- Care Plans

Your request will get the staff's complete and undivided attention, because few people outside the health-care system would be familiar with these items. Any nervousness on the staff's part might be attributable to the fact that all the documents haven't been properly completed, as often happens. Because you seem to know a lot about medical records, you'll likely be asked what you are looking for, and perhaps even "What kind of work do you do?" Persist, politely, but firmly. If you have the legal right to look at the patient's records, the staff must produce them for you.

Weight and Skin Charts

The MDS, RAP sheet and modules, and care plans are not the end of the nurses' documentation. Weight and skin charts are also important monitoring tools.

Weight Chart

From the weight chart (Figure 15), you can see that measurements were made once a month until August, when they were made once a week.

HERITAGE HARBOUR HEALTH & REHABILITATION CENTER

MONTHLY & WEEKLY WEIGHTS

YEAR 2000

MONTH	DATE	TYPE OF SCALE	WEIGHT	CHANGE +/-	REWEIGHT	% CHANGE	WEEK 1	WEEK 2	WEEK 3	WEEK 4	WEEK 5
January						%30D %90D %180D					
February						%30D %90D %180D					
March						%30D %90D %180D					
April	4/26		118.8			%30D %90D %180D					
May	5/16		113			%30D %90D %180D	5/26 111.8				
June	6/5		104			%30D %90D %180D					
July	7/10		99.4			%30D %90D %180D					
August	8/3		92.8			%30D %90D %180D	8/10 90.2	8/17 91.2	8/25 91.2		
September	9/7		91.8			%30D %90D %180D	9/14 88.6				
October						%30D %90D %180D					
November						%30D %90D %180D					
December						%30D %90D %180D					

RESIDENT Watters, Mary   MR# 00216   MD _____

Figure 15: Monthly and weekly weight charts show weight trends.

No Plan Developed to Address Nutritional Status

A physician's order dated May 30, 2000 documented the resident was to receive one can of Boost Nutritional Supplement two times a day. There was no nutritional documentation in the resident's record after June 19, 2000. A physician's order dated July 10, 2000 documented the resident's diet was to be changed to pureed. A review of the resident's comprehensive care plan dated April 24, 2000 which documented, "(Resident #29) does not appear responsive to environment. Needs environmental stimulation and pleasurable experiences." The staff approaches included, "Serve favorite foods when possible and allow time to savor taste. Describe food before it is offered." There was no plan of care which addressed the resident's nutritional status, weight loss and potential for further weight loss.

– State survey, Tucson, Arizona, July 15, 2000

Changes in weight are an important sign in the elderly, so it is critical to monitor the weight chart carefully. Weight loss is generally the problem, but weight gain can also be serious. For example, a gain of 10 pounds in a one-week period might indicate that the patient is retaining fluid because of a heart or kidney condition. If the patient continues to retain fluid at this rate, the next likely step would be acute shortness of breath culminating in a trip to the hospital for treatment of congestive heart failure or kidney disease. With the patient whose case Figure 15 concerns, inadequate fluid and nutritional intake caused the weight loss. The patient was not on a pureed diet, was having difficulty swallowing, and she probably wasn't receiving sufficient assistance in eating.

Weight loss is often a function of food intake. Of course, food being expensive and nursing homes being businesses, it shouldn't surprise you to learn that one medical equipment company tried to market a system to help nursing homes reduce food costs. The scheme calculated the calories needed by a patient at rest in bed and added about 10 percent to arrive at a figure representing the total calories needed by the patient.

The "win-win" formula this sadistic group developed would have saved a nursing home money by reducing the outlay for food – and the patients would supposedly be healthier because they'd be that much closer to their ideal body weight. The idea here would have been

Patient Isn't Repositioned and Pressure Sores Result

A physician's order dated 03/31/00 documented that she had a skin tear in the middle of buttocks. . . .Clean with normal saline and apply Neosporin ointment, cover with dry dressing 2 times daily.

A care plan dated 04/30/00 (1 month later) documented the skin tear was healing slowly. Continue treatment as ordered and notify the physician if the treatment was ineffective. A care plan related to the risk of pressure sore breakdown documented that Resident #7 was to be repositioned every 2 hours.

On 05/01/00 Resident #7 was observed to be lying in bed on her back at the following times: 9:45 a.m., 10:30 a.m., 11:15 a.m., 12:30 p.m., 1:00 p.m., 1:30 p.m., and 3:00 p.m.

Resident #7's "skin tear" was observed on 05/01/00 at 3 p.m. with the Director of Nurses (DON). The DON discovered three Stage 2 pressure areas left buttock, right buttock and in the crease in the middle of the buttocks (where the original skin tear had occurred.) An egg crate mattress was observed on Resident #7's bed. The DON confirmed that egg crate mattresses provided no pressure reduction and that Neosporin was not the treatment of choice for pressure sores.

On 05/01/00 a new physician's treatment order was obtained for one (the middle Stage 2 pressure area) of the three pressure areas. This pressure area was measured as 1.5 x .05 cm.

As of 05/03/00 at 11:30 a.m. there was no documented evidence that the physician was notified of the other two pressure areas, that treatment orders were obtained or the pressure areas on the left and right buttock were assessed.

– State survey, Sacramento, California, May 15, 2000

to tell a 200-pound patient her ideal body weight was 125 pounds and that the object was to help her get there. This clever solution to reducing food costs didn't catch on, but that a company even tried to peddle it demonstrates why you must constantly monitor your loved one's care to make sure that finances aren't dictating it rather than medicine.

Skin Chart

The Pressure Area Record (Figure 16), or skin chart, is the next item that you'll want to check. As you can see, this skin chart for the coccyx describes the size, color, and drainage of the bedsore and lists various questions relevant to treatment. This sheet needs to be updated and read on a routine basis. If you can't find it in the chart, ask for it. Bedsores are mostly preventable and are an indication of poor nursing care. The stages of bedsores range from I to IV, with IV, the worst, being down to bone level. See Appendix E for illustrations and descriptions of bedsores, which are also called pressure sores or pressure areas.

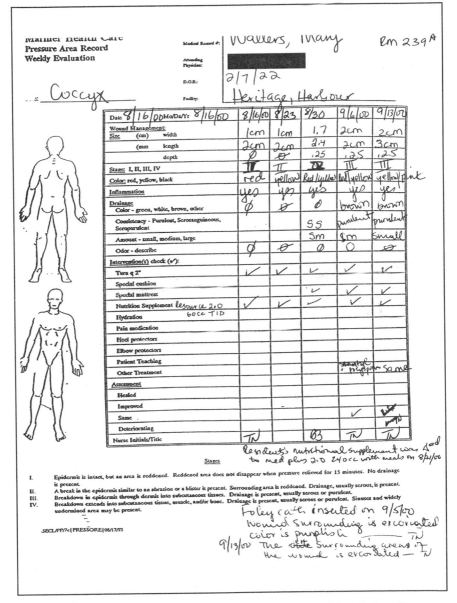

Figure 16: Pressure Area Record – evaluation and description of bedsore on the coccyx.

MARS and TARS

Keep in mind that as of this point none of the documentation we've reviewed means that anything has actually been done for Mom. Documentation that treatment has been provided rests with the nurses and can be found in MARS and TARS reports.

MARS

Let's start by looking at the MARS (Medication Administration Record System). At first blush this report (Figure 17) might appear confusing, but analyzing it isn't as mysterious a process as you might think. The patient's name is recorded at the bottom, as are the dates for this reporting period, from 5/1/00 to 5/31/00. In the left column are the names of the drugs to be given. The amounts and concentrations are listed, but ignore that for now.

The next column has the date 4/26/00. That is the date the order started. Underneath that date, in the time column, you will either see the notation "PRN," which means as needed, or a time for the drug to be given, such as 8:30 a.m. As you read across the form, note the little numbers that range from 1 to 28. These numbers correspond to the day of the month. If you see a mark in the box below the number 12, you know that that drug was given on the 12th day of May.

A new MARS is started for each month, which is why you need to look for the range of dates at the bottom. The little marks you see in the boxes are not just the letter "X," but rather the initials of the person who administered the medication. This is how you can identify the responsible party.

The straight lines you see indicate nothing was done relative to this order during that time. Entries for KCL, a drug that replaces potassium, which is important in heart function, shows that administration of the drug did not start until May 27.

To avoid confusion or wrong entries later, the nurses place a line through the previous days for which there was no order. When specific times are listed for a drug to be administered, you will be able to determine the day and time it was given and the person who administered it. If you see a 4 p.m. dose checked off at 10 a.m., it's obvious the record has been falsified. This little move is a classic, particularly with tube feedings and other such regularly scheduled procedures, so watch out for it.

It's a good idea to get in the habit of looking at the MARS. This document is also referred to as the "Kardex" – as in "Please let me see my mother's Kardex." Are the orders you discussed with the doctor recorded here? If not, you can be sure whatever you've requested will not be done.

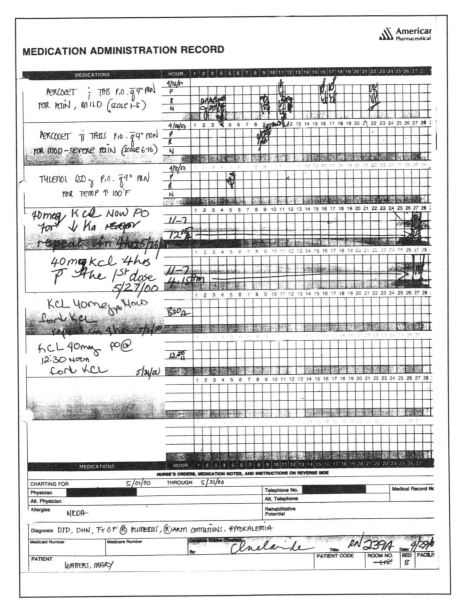

Figure 17: MARS – Medication Administration Record System report for 5/1/2000 through 5/31/2000.

TARS

The MARS is for medication, but other items need to be recorded. These are charted in the TARS (Treatment Administration Record System). As you can see from the sample (Figure 18) provided, nurses chart things in exactly the same manner as on the MARS. Let's look at one entry near the bottom: Foley Care Q Shift and PRN. Look at the initials, dates, and so on. You will see that the staff members have documented care of the

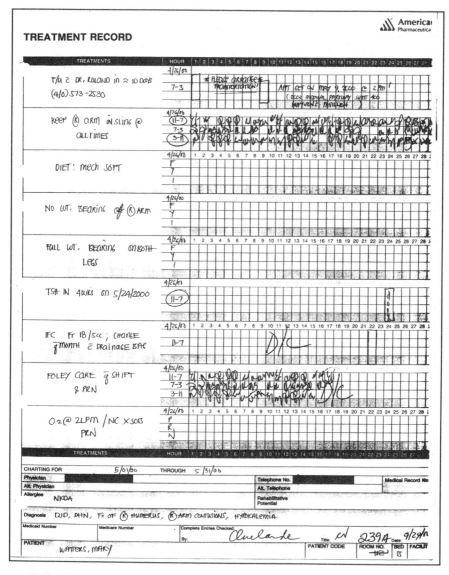

Figure 18: *TARS – Treatment Administration Record System report for 5/1/2000 through 5/31/2000.*

urinary catheter on May 16 for two shifts and on May 17 for one shift. At that point, the service was D/C, or discontinued.

But wait a minute. Take a look at Figure 19, which contains the nursing note (second from bottom) for 05/15/2000 at 6 p.m.: "IFC pulled out as per M.D.'s order." It was not possible to provide Foley catheter care on 05/16 and 05/17, as documented in the TARS, when the device was removed on 05/15. A finding such as this puts the entire record in doubt. How can you believe what the caregivers are saying when they have lied in the medical record? This may sound like nitpicking, but this discrepancy cannot be brushed aside, because the falsification occurred over two days and involved more than one person. What else did the patient not receive that her records indicated she had?

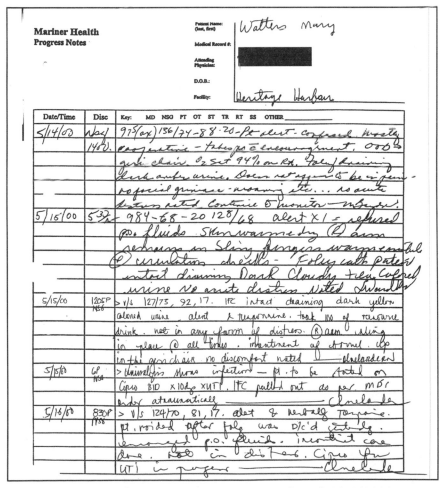

Figure 19: Nursing notes for 5/14/2000 through 5/16/2000.

7
CONSULTATIONS and LABORATORY DATA

In addition to orders and physician and nursing notes, medical records also contain reports from consulting physicians and laboratories. It is not uncommon for the primary medical doctor to request assistance in the diagnosis and treatment of specific problems outside his area of expertise. Common examples would include podiatry, ophthalmology, and dentistry.

Normally, the physician will request in writing an opinion regarding the management of the patient. Following examination, the consulting physician or dentist will provide a consultation note in the medical chart that generally follows the SOAP format. Reviewing consultation notes is worth the effort, so you can be sure that the suggestions have been reviewed and implemented by your physician.

Consultation Report

Figure 20 is a typical nursing home consultation report, in this case concerning fractures in the patient's pelvic area and the deterioration of her right shoulder. The key items are the diagnosis and the recommendations for treatment and follow-up. Notice that the attending physician who requested the consultation did not complete the reason for it (on the lines following Report Requested/Regarding) and did not sign the form (on the line above "Report"). These omissions could have had several undesirable consequences, not the least of which would have been the specialist's overlooking something important or prescribing a drug for which the patient is allergic. Additionally, a consultation can only be billed if there has been a formal request by a physician. This can be accomplished in several ways, but the best one is have a signed consultation request.

In a situation such as the one in Figure 20, the family should make sure that the specialist's orders have been transferred to the physician's order sheet and the MARS and TARS, and that the nursing care plan has been updated. Remember, if the specialist's recommendations are not in the orders, they will not be carried out. The specialist recommended keeping the right arm in a sling. If the family found that this was not being done, it would want to ask why.

Laboratory Report

Laboratory information might include blood and urine test results, usually found in one section of the chart. Fortunately, most laboratories include the normal range for each of the values because they can vary

Figure 20: Consultation report.

from lab to lab. When you notice an abnormal laboratory result, you should find a corresponding note in the physician's area that addresses the identified problem. If you are not sure of the significance of an abnormal result, you should ask your physician to explain it to you.

The lab report in Figure 21 deals in part with the kidney. It shows a blood urea nitrogen (BUN) level that is borderline acceptable and an elevated glucose level. The creatinine level is normal. The BUN and creatinine levels are indicative of the kidney's health. When the creatinine level is normal and the BUN is high, the patient is dehydrated. In this patient's chart, the physician circled the BUN value because he realized that though the lab did not flag the condition as abnormal it was a possible indication of dehydration.

Note that the nursing home stamped the report at the bottom to show when the report was received and when the M.D. was notified. This effectively shifts the responsibility for the next decision to the physician.

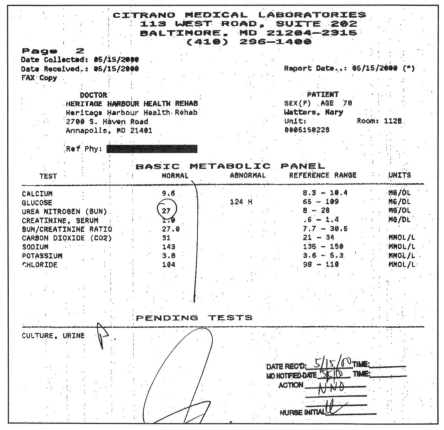

Figure 21: Laboratory report.

8
THE "THREE-BY-FIVES" METHOD

Orders, notes, MARS, TARS, MDS, RAP, ICP – we've given you quite
a bit of background. You're probably asking yourself, "How am I ever
going to remember all of this?" Well, it turns out that physicians have
exactly the same problem when trying to remember their patients' conditions. One way they address the issue is by using three-by-five-inch
index cards. The cards are especially popular with resident physicians,
who are doctors in training. During morning rounds, the residents discuss the problems of various patients and potential solutions to those
problems. The three-by-fives allow a resident to present a patient's situation concisely.

Creating Your Own Three-by-Fives
Creating your own three-by-five (Figure 22) is fairly straightforward.
Create one card every month or so. Remember that the purpose of the
card is to remind you of the patient's conditions and what you need
to check.

As you can see from the example provided, the three-by-fives outline
the basic situation:

- Who are the responsible parties?
- Why is the patient in the nursing home?
- What are the goals of treatment?
- What plans have been made to address the problems and
  reach the goals?
- Are the plans being implemented?
- Are the plans working and if not what is being done to
  change them?
- What do you want done for the patient?
- What do you see, smell, hear, and feel?
- What problems have you noticed, who have you
  contacted about them, and what is being done about them?

FRONT OF CARD

Name: _____   Room Number: _____ Phone: _____

Doctor: _____   Phone: _____

Nurse: _____   (7 a.m.– 3 p.m.; 3–11 p.m.; 11 p.m.–7 a.m.)

List of patient's problems: stroke, diabetes, pneumonia
Goals: weight gain, increased mobility, decreased pain, and so on
What you want done: special diet, pain medication, sleeping aid

What is staff doing today to meet goals? To find out, check order sheets, medical and treatment records, nurses notes, progress notes.

What should they be doing? To find out, check care plans, progress notes, consultation notes, physical-therapy plans, dietician's notes, RAP summary.

What should you check? Look at weight, eating and drinking, mouth hygiene, skin condition, comfort, smells; look under sheets, at heels, lower back, and arms and legs for sores and tears.

BACK OF CARD

DATE	PROBLEM	WHO WAS TOLD/ WHAT WAS DONE?
03/02/02	foul odor, not clean, no water	Sandy, got water, changed diaper
03/05/02	foul odor, not changed again	Sandy and Administrator /promises
04/05/02	skin ulcer, dirty diaper	nursing director, doctor, treatment
04/07/02	skin ulcer worse, fever	moved to hospital ER

Figure 22: *A three-by-five card will help you remember what you need to check.*

Tip: Try to stick with only one three-by-five card per month. This will help you to concentrate only on the important tasks of identifying problems, and finding out what the planned treatments and goals will be, and evaluating the success of treatments.

Don't worry if you don't understand everything you're noting. And don't feel bad about asking a lot of questions or taking staff members' time, or pointing out discrepancies you notice in the medical record. The home took the money; it's the job of the staff to provide proper care. Your job is to protect your loved one, get the best care possible, and prevent Mom or Dad from falling victim to the nursing home's bottom line.

9
ACT BEFORE IT'S TOO LATE

A nursing home is a document-centered universe. Everything revolves around documentation – the recording of information, the reviewing of it, and the archiving of it. As a concerned friend or family member you need to penetrate and understand this world if you are to improve the care your loved one receives. In this book we have provided you with the knowledge and tools you need to take action. Do not sit back and hope things will get better. As a user of our site from Arlington, Texas, related in a recent e-mail, you need to act before it's too late:

> I just wanted to let you know I followed through with my complaint on the lack of care for my friend that died. I filed a complaint with the state; the investigator called me and said I should have called when he [the friend] was a patient at the nursing home I was complaining about. Although she checked their records, they did not match what I had told her. He had lost 60 pounds – they documented a loss of only 8 pounds! They would not check with his doctor or the hospital he was taken to. What an eye-opening experience for me! You are correct. I should have gained access to the medical records while he was still alive.

Everyone in the nursing home is documenting everything they do or say they have done. Don't be the odd person out. Make your own notes and communicate often – and in writing – with the home's administrator and director of nursing. Keep copies of everything.

This really is a matter of life and death.

10
GENERAL WORKSHEET

If you become greatly concerned about the care your loved one is receiving, with the General Worksheet provided in this section you can monitor patient care and the condition of the home. The Staff Worksheet in the next section will identify the strengths and weaknesses of the nursing home's staff and procedures. Collecting and analyzing this data will make it easier for you to articulate your areas of concern and will help you to keep the staff focused on the problems you or the doctors, nurses, or other staff members have observed. The data will also support your complaints should this be required. Full-size reproductions of both charts are provided at the end of the book – you may find it helpful to refer to them as you read through this section. Later you can make photocopies of the charts to track care issues and note your concerns.

The General Worksheet deals with the condition of the patient and the home and covers nine main areas:

- Flow-sheet data
- General services
- Staffing
- Safety
- Grooming
- Specialized services
- Complaints
- Problems
- Drug Therapy

At the very top of the page is space to list the month. Across the top of the page are squares in which you should write the particular day you are making your documentation. These columns run to the right of the word "Day." There are 15 columns, so the worksheet can easily be used in either bi-weekly or monthly format. Create a separate general worksheet for each period you choose. This will allow you to track each item by month and day so that you can monitor trends over time.

The setup we have developed here is very similar to that of MARS and TARS reports. In the left column of each of these sections you'll see an area or item of interest. Below that you will find the specific things to monitor in that group.

Flow Sheets

Flow sheets are the forms that staff members fill out to track a specific activity or problem over time. By doing the same, you will be better able to keep track of the results the staff has noted and posted about weight changes and skin condition, for example.

GENERAL WORKSHEET Month: Day ▶							
FLOW SHEETS							
WEIGHT (on admission: _____ lbs.)							
VITAL SIGNS							
SKIN SHEETS AND LOG							
coccyx							
left hip							
left heel							
right hip							
right heel							
turn and position							
other							
DIET							
food intake							
fluid intake / output							
water available / clean cup							

General Worksheet: Flow sheet.

Weight

The first example is the patient's weight. Write the admission weight in the blank space on the "Weight" line. Under each subsequent date on which weight has been checked you can either enter the weight, or just a symbol to indicate that the staff has checked it and whether it has gone up or down. For example, you might wish to use "+" or "–" signs. The best strategy, though, is to enter the weight as recorded that day. This will eliminate confusion about any increases or decreases you have observed.

Increases or decreases in weight are important to monitor. Though increases are sometimes seen in patients who enter the facility malnourished, large increases during a short period of time generally reflect water retention. The usual causes include heart and kidney disease. If the retention is significant, swelling of the ankles often occurs. You can easily confirm this. Press on the skin over the ankle or shinbone. If doing so leaves an indentation, this is called pitting edema, or swelling. The farther up the shin or the larger the ankle diameter, the worse the problem likely is. If you observe this condition, point it out to the doctor. He or she may not have looked under the covers. Another way to monitor swelling in the leg is to use a tape measure and actually measure the diameter of the leg. The measurements should all be made at the same point, say, 4 inches below the center of the kneecap.

The more common problem is weight loss, the causes of which include difficulty with chewing or swallowing, mouth pain, improper diet, and inadequate food and water. The actual amount of weight gained or loss should be noted, and in percentages – for example, 5 percent in the last 30 days, or 10 percent in the last 180 days. These are the standards used in the Resident Assessment Protocol. The patient's weight should be measured at least every 30 days and more frequently as indicated.

Vital Signs

The vital-signs flow sheets record the patient's blood pressure, temperature, pulse, and respiratory rate.

Blood pressure is expressed as one number over the other, such as 120/80. The top number, or systolic, refers to the pressure of the blood during a heartbeat, and the lower number, or diastolic, refers to the pressure between heartbeats. Both numbers are significant. The normal blood pressure is between 120 and 129mmHg systolic and 80 and 84 mmHg diastolic (mmHg stands for millimeters of mercury, which is used in the instrument to measure blood pressure.) In a petite person, for example, it could easily be 95/60. The normal upper range ends at about 135/90.

A normal **pulse,** or heart rate, is about 80 beats per minute. Some drugs, though, cause the heart to beat only 60 times per minute. Much lower than this in a nonathlete is reason for concern and evaluation.

Resting heart rates above 100 are considered abnormal and are usually the consequence of dehydration, heart problems, or stressors such as pain or infection. Some medications also cause an increased heart rate.

The normal **temperature** is 98.6 degrees Fahrenheit. If the temperature is above 100.4 Fahrenheit it is considered a fever, and someone needs to determine why the temperature is elevated. Two common causes among nursing home residents are urinary tract infections (UTIs) and pneumonia. A UTI is very common when the patient has an in-dwelling urinary catheter.

The normal **respiratory rate,** or breathing rate, is about 14 breaths per minute. Breathing patterns are important and beyond the scope of this manual, but if you notice the respiratory rate falling to 10, then 8, then 6, and then 4 breaths per minute, immediate attention is required because respiratory arrest is imminent. Cardiac arrest is next, because the heart needs oxygen to work. Death may follow.

A patient breathing 20, then 25, then 30, and then 40 times per minute also constitutes an emergency situation. Patients breathe at a rapid rate because they are either not getting enough oxygen or need to expel a lot of carbon dioxide. In both cases, a respiratory rate of 35 or 40 times per minute cannot be sustained for very long because of the great energy required. Sudden respiratory arrest can result, or a slowing of the breathing rate, with an increase in carbon dioxide levels in the blood, which affects the brain, and the subsequent loss of consciousness. This is then followed by death secondary to full respiratory arrest or cardiac arrest or both.

Look to see if the staff is recording pulse and respiratory rates. Are they always the same? If this is the case, you have reason to become a little suspicious. You can check the pulse and respiratory rate at the bedside with a watch with a second hand. Feel for the patient's pulse in the wrist. Count the number of beats in 60 seconds and you're done.

Also keep track of the pulse's regularity. If it is irregularly irregular, then the patient most likely has atrial fibrillation, or, simply, an irregular force or rhythm to the heartbeat. You'll be able to detect this easily enough because you will not be able to guess when the next pulse is coming. This condition makes estimating a pulse rate more of a challenge. If you notice this condition, mention it to the nurse or the doctor, though one or both should have detected it well before you do.

You can check respiration the same way. Just look for the chest expanding and contracting. But make sure you measure a complete up-and-down cycle. For example, if you start measuring when the chest is expanded, you count the next breath when the chest expands again, not when the chest contracts. Your numbers should be fairly close to the staff's. Note if the breathing is regular, deep, shallow, or if there is a pattern. Don't tell your mom you are counting her breathing rate. This may cause it to be higher than normal. One technique is to hold her wrist as if checking the pulse, but actually count the respirations.

Skin

Bedsores, also known as decubitus ulcers or pressure sores, are among the most preventable problems in nursing homes, but once present can be difficult to treat. The stages of skin ulcers range from Stage I to Stage IV. A Stage I ulcer is a reddened area of skin that overlies a prominent bone, like the hip or heel, and does not disappear when pressure is relieved. Stage II is when there is a superficial break in the skin like a blister or abrasion. Stage III indicates a much deeper ulcer. At Stage IV you can see bone or muscle. Nursing home staffs are extremely diligent about examining patients on admission. They don't want to get blamed for bedsores that did not occur at their facility. After admission, however, diligence sometimes falters.

Check to see that a skin chart exists, what if anything has been noted, and whether entries are made regularly. The most common areas where bedsores occur are the tailbone, the hip, and the heel. Examine these areas yourself. If you see something, mark it down, and see whether the staff's records reflect what you have observed. Skin tears, abrasions, and related matters can also be addressed on this sheet. If the patient has restricted mobility, check the TARS to be sure the patient is being turned every two hours. If you are finding bedsores that have not been recorded or addressed by the staff, it's time to take a photograph.

Diet

Dietary flow sheets should indicate what portion of the food for each meal has been eaten – for example, 25 percent at breakfast and 75 percent at dinner. Review the charts with the dietician and ask if the patient is consuming enough calories. At some homes, the percentage of food left uneaten is charted. Ask what is being recorded.

Fluid intake and output is also important, especially in someone who is dehydrated. A kidney that is functioning normally will put out 500cc of urine per day even if there is no water intake. This is how a patient can become dehydrated. When the kidney output starts to fall below 500cc per day it is an early indication of kidney failure. If the cause is inadequate fluid intake, the condition can usually be reversed with ease.

Keeping track of urine output is especially easy if the patient has a urinary catheter in place. In this situation, request that the output be charted as well as the input. Bedridden patients not receiving sufficient water and food are well on their way to getting bedsores. Make sure that water and other liquids are available to the patient in an easy-to-reach cup. Also, make sure the cup is clean and changed regularly. If Styrofoam cups are used, mark the date on the bottom of the cup. The patient should receive a new cup every day or so. Look for growth of mold in the cup, or curdling if milk products are used.

General Services

The items in this realm are self-explanatory. You don't need to monitor them daily, but they are worth inspecting every week or two. Place

GENERAL WORKSHEET Month: Day ▶							
GENERAL SERVICES							
LINEN							
bed changed							
clothes changed and clean							
diaper changed							
towels available and clean							
other							
PEST CONTROL							
BATHROOM							
soap in dispenser							
towels in dispenser							
toilet paper							
bedpan clean and available							
staff washes hands							

General Worksheet: General services.

a checkmark in the box corresponding to the date you made your observations. If any items are not to your liking, let the staff know what you want done about the problem. Pest control is important, because with so much food being delivered up and down the hallways and into individual rooms, bug infestation is always a possibility. Cases have been reported of nursing homes being overcome with fire ants, causing bedridden patients much distress. If you notice bugs or other pests, take a photograph.

Staffing

This is another area that need not be monitored daily. Talk with the director of nursing to establish how many of each type of practitioner are on the floor during each shift. Also ask how many patients are on the floor. From this information you can calculate the number of hours per day available for each patient's care. Staffing is an important issue. Some patients require more care than others, and some homes take on more serious cases than others, but according to a Congressional report published in 2000, there is very strong evidence that residents in nursing homes with higher staff-to-patient ratios receive a better quality of care than at facilities with lower ones.

GENERAL WORKSHEET Month: Day ►								
STAFFING								
REGISTERED NURSE								
LICENSED PRACTICAL NURSE								
NURSING ASSISTANT								
CERTIFIED MEDICAL ASSISTANT								

General Worksheet: Staffing.

Safety

As you evaluate the safety-related items, place a check in the appropriate date box if all is well. The feet can be a problem area. Footboards are devices placed at the foot of the bed to keep the sheets off the patient's feet and prevent the patient from getting contractures (shortening of the tendons). When these occur in the foot area, the Achilles tendon becomes shorter and the toes point down. As you can imagine, this condition would make walking nearly impossible. Passive range-of-motion exercise by the staff as well as the footboard will help prevent the problem.

If the patient spends large amounts of time in bed, make sure he or she has adequate padding on the bed itself and the heels of the feet, which helps to ward off bedsores. Padding the hands is also important for patients with contractures of the wrists and fingers. Without this padding, a patient's fingernails can cut into the palms of the hands. Also, make sure the call button is within reach, that it works, and that the patient is able to use it. If restraints are present, make sure they have been ordered by the doctor, and find out under what circumstances. You don't want your relative tied to a chair for six hours straight just because it is convenient for the staff. The only rational use of restraints is to prevent injury to the patient. If they are being used, find out why and make sure they are installed correctly.

GENERAL WORKSHEET Month: Day ▶							
SAFETY							
BEDRAILS							
available / working / being used							
NO SKID SLIPPERS							
available							
in use if appropriate							
ROOM TEMPERATURE							
LIGHTING							
ELECTRIC BED							
PADS: BED / HEELS / FEET / HANDS							
FOOT BOARD: CONTRACTURES							
CALL BUTTON / working / in reach							
RESTRAINT USE							
proper medical order							
used appropriately							
used properly							

General Worksheet: Safety.

Safety Issues Not Properly Addressed

Nursing notes on 6/4/00 at 0400, stated the resident was at high risk for falls. On 6/9/00 at 0545, the resident was found on the floor of his room, beside his bed, in front of his wheelchair. Subsequent to the incident, the record indicated the resident was placed on "falling stars" program, but there was no in depth assessment related to the cause of the 6/9/00 incident. The fall RAP module assessment summary was left blank on the 6/9/00 RAI.

— State survey, Cheyenne, Wyoming, June 17, 2000

Inaccuracy in MDS

Review of the resident's medical record revealed that the most recently completed MDS dated 1/6/99 contained the following inaccuracy.

Section P4 indicated the use of a trunk restraint daily. Observation of the resident on each day of the survey and interview of the nursing staff on 3/11/99 revealed that the resident did not use a trunk restraint.

– State survey, Hagerstown, Maryland, March 17, 1999

Grooming

Grooming issues are easier to identify than medical ones, but you need to monitor them. Having a checklist will help you identify problems. In addition, it provides a record that can be reviewed with staff members so that you can help them maintain the appropriate focus.

GENERAL WORKSHEET Month: Day ▶						
GROOMING						
HAIR						
washed						
fixed						
falling out						
texture						
ORAL HYGIENE						
debris in mouth						
evidence of toothbrush use						
bleeding of gums						
bad breath						
broken or missing teeth						
missings fillings / caps / bridges						
dentures available						
dentures fit						
dentures clean						
SKIN						
washed						
clean						
TOENAILS						
FINGERNAILS						

General Worksheet: Grooming.

Specialized Services

Specialized services include not only items unique to a given patient, but also those that are important for all patients. Items such as activities and sleeping aids are listed under specialized services because they require specific physician's orders. Activities might include exercise, passive range of motion, being moved from a bed to a chair, or art therapy. Effective pain relief cannot be stressed enough. Be sure you know how pain relief is being evaluated and monitored. Patients may not be able to verbalize their discomfort, so the care plans should take this into account. The patient should not have to ask for pain relief – it should be offered on a regular basis. Narcotics can increase the likelihood of constipation and fecal impaction, but this is preventable. Check to see if stool softeners are needed. In the event of diarrhea, the cause must be determined and a plan of treatment prescribed, or significant bedsores will result.

A urinary catheter can be necessary but it is sometimes used for the convenience of the staff. An in-dwelling catheter – one that stays in all the time – is apt to cause bleeding in the bladder through irritation. But, more importantly, it can be a source of infection, some of which can become life threatening. Check the tension of the catheter. The catheter should be anchored to the thigh if possible to prevent excessive motion. There should be enough slack in the catheter between the thigh and the urethra to allow for movement. You can imagine how uncomfortable this would be if it were pulling all the time.

For men, improperly secured in-dwelling catheters may result in pressure that can cause ulcerations on the head of the penis at the urethra. This is preventable. If you notice cloudy, malodorous urine, or urine with blood, bring this to the staff's attention. If the catheter will be replaced, ask if an anesthesia of some sort will be used. The answer "none" is not appropriate. With the exception of an allergy to the topical anesthetic, there is no reason why lidocaine jelly cannot not be used in place of K-Y lubricating jelly or only Betadine, a topical microbicide often used in this situation. The placing of an in-dwelling catheter involves washing the area with Betadine (if the patient is not allergic to iodine), and then draping the sterile field. The catheter is removed from the sterile packing and lubricant is applied to the catheter prior to placement. Lidocaine jelly, which is a local anesthetic, is not often part of the standard kit.

An even kinder method would involve the injection of lidocaine jelly into the urethra, male or female, using a syringe without a needle. At this point, the entire urethra would be numb and the additional lidocaine jelly on the catheter would serve as lubricant. Staff people tend not to want to use lidocaine jelly because it is not part of the kit. It has to be sent from the pharmacy, which requires a physician's order. For the staff members, it comes down to their time versus the patient's pain. Absent your intervention, your loved one might lose. Occasionally, urinary catheters are used on a one-time basis, to obtain a sterile urine sample for a culture, for instance. The suggestions for pain relief above apply in this situation too.

The other items listed, such as activities, sleeping aids, pain relief, and the identification of depression, are important as part of the entire process of providing care.

GENERAL WORKSHEET Month: Day ▶							
SPECIALIZED SERVICES							
CATHETER CARE							
is it needed							
changed regularly							
no tension or pulling							
urinary bag emptied							
no sediment in bag or tubing							
smell, color of urine normal							
ACTIVITIES							
SLEEPING AIDS							
EFFECTIVE PAIN RELIEF							
DEPRESSION							
indications							
treatment							
BOWEL ROUTINE							

General Worksheet: Specialized services.

Complaints

This is where you note your complaints and check off the date. Keep a separate log for all your complaints, with detailed notes on what you saw, with whom you spoke about the problem, and whether or not you filed a letter. If you take photographs of any medical condition that concerns you, such as a bedsore, document the date they were taken.

GENERAL WORKSHEET Month: Day ➤								
COMPLAINTS								
1								
2								
3								
4								
5								
6								

General Worksheet: Complaints.

Problems

On this part of the worksheet, you should list the patient's problems. These might include weight loss, heart difficulties, stroke, abnormal lab values, diabetes, hypertension, or bedsores. Note the date these problems were first recorded and when they were resolved. Under the days of the month, you can enter "S" for start of a problem and "E" to indicate the problem has ended.

You can make up an initial problem list by looking at the physician's notes and by examining the Resident Assessment Protocol (RAP). The nurses' care plans should also list the patient's problems. As you review the care plan or other charts, add to your list any problems you haven't already noted. For each problem, make up a Problem Worksheet so you can monitor the staff's evaluation, assessment, and care plan. Lapses in attention over time will become immediately obvious, your indication that that you need to refocus the team.

GENERAL WORKSHEET Month: Day ➤								
PROBLEM (START DATE)								
1								
2								
3								
4								
5								

General Worksheet: Problems.

Drug Therapy

The last part of the General Worksheet deals with drugs and supplements, allowing you to track medications that have been ordered and whether or not they have been administered. You can get the list of drugs prescribed for the patient from the physician's order sheets. Then ask to see the MARS and TARS reports, in which you should find verification that the drugs have actually been administered. (If you see at 10 a.m. that an order for a drug to be given at 3 p.m. has already been charted, this is clearly a problem. File a written complaint, for this is record falsification. Do not accept an answer like "we always chart in advance." The records should always reflect what has actually been done, not what might be done in the future.)

On the worksheet, record the name of the drug and the number of times per day it is to be given. Here are a few abbreviations: q.d. = once per day; q.h.s. = hour of sleep; b.i.d. = twice a day; t.i.d. = three times a day; q.i.d. = four times a day; q12h means every 12 hours; and q8 or q8h means every eight hours.

If you read something like "Percocet 1 tab q4h prn pain," this means the staff is supposed to give the patient one tablet of Percocet every four hours as needed for pain. Find out how the staff is evaluating the patient for the "prn" (as needed) order. Remember that patients aren't always able to request pain relief. A better order would be, "Evaluate patient for pain every four hours while awake, chart results, and dispense Tylenol two tablets for mild pain, Tylenol #3 two tablets for moderate pain, Percocet one or two tablets for severe pain." This places the burden squarely where it belongs, on the staff personnel who are being paid to care for the patient.

GENERAL WORKSHEET Month: Day ▶						
DRUG THERAPY (NAME, T.I.D., B.I.D., etc.)						
1						
2						
3						
4						
5						
6						
7						
8						

General Worksheet: Drug therapy.

11
STAFF WORKSHEET

The Staff Worksheet will help you to monitor how the staff resolves specific problems the patient has and to keep track of the therapies that are prescribed.

Physician Notes

Let's begin with the physician (progress) notes. With a checkmark, indicate the days on which the doctor made notes. For the problem under consideration, did he or she make entries about symptoms? Were there objective findings? Is there evidence that an assessment or plan was developed for this problem? If specific plans were made, were new orders written? If so, do the MARS and TARS reports show that they have been implemented? Mark your chart accordingly.

You may find in many instances in which you have checked off that the doctor wrote a progress note but have no evidence the specific problem was addressed. Depending on the situation, this may be acceptable. Often, doctors only address problems that appear to be changing in some way. For example, if the problem is control of the blood sugar level in a patient with diabetes and it is stable and well controlled, there may be no entry. Your job is to make sure that someone has checked to see the condition really is under control. If you don't think this has happened, you should ask the nurse, the attending physician, or both.

STAFF WORKSHEET Month: Day ➤							
PHYSICIAN NOTES							
SYMPTOMS							
OBJECTIVE FINDINGS							
ASSESSMENT							
PLAN							
evidence in MARS							
evidence in TARS							

Staff Worksheet: Physician notes.

Nursing Notes

The notes nurses take are usually the best in the chart, especially when compared with the doctor's notes. Look in the contemporaneous notes for information about the problem you're tracking. (In facilities

STAFF WORKSHEET Month:	Day ▶								
NURSING NOTES									
SYMPTOMS									
OBJECTIVE FINDINGS									
ASSESSMENT									
MDS									
RAP									
CARE PLANS									
evidence in MARS									
evidence in TARS									

Staff Worksheet: Nursing notes.

that "chart by exception" – which only document circumstances that fall outside the care plan, such as a patient falling out of bed – the notes will not cover every problem.) Examine the care plan to ensure that the problem has been identified, a goal has been defined, and a treatment plan has been devised. Later, look for evidence that the staff has evaluated the treatment's effectiveness. You will often find such evidence in the minimum data set (MDS) and on the resident assessment protocol (RAP). The success of any care plan is directly related to its implementation, though, so next check the MARS and TARS to find out if it has actually been instituted.

Catheter Bag Placement Causes Problems for Patient

The resident had an in-dwelling catheter in place. The catheter bag was lying on his bed. The resident's foot of bed had been elevated and the catheter bag placed next to his feet. When the surveyor asked the resident and his family member about the catheter bag they replied, "An aide put the bag in his bed because she tried to get him up. That was awhile ago about 15 to 20 minutes." The resident stated "My sheet was full of blood because yesterday afternoon before my shower, my catheter tubing got caught in the sling of the maxi lift." This was verified by staff and an incident report had been filled out. . . .

– State survey, Ludington, Michigan, September 15, 2000

Other Providers and Complaints

Similar audits of the work of other providers should be conducted, including dieticians and occupational, speech, and physical therapists. Also include any specialists such as ophthalmologists, orthopedists, dentists, and podiatrists. After these items, you can keep a record of complaints and add notes. At the end of the month, you should be able to look back at each worksheet you have completed and identify who addressed the problem. If you see many blank spaces, you should ask yourself why.

STAFF WORKSHEET Month: Day ➤								
THERAPY (OT, PT, SPEECH, DIETICIAN)								
PROVIDER:								
evidence in MARS and TARS								
PROVIDER:								
evidence in MARS and TARS								
PROVIDER:								
evidence in MARS and TARS								
OTHER THERAPY IN ORDERS:								
evidence in MARS and TARS								
COMPLAINTS / NOTES								
1								
2								
3								
4								

Staff Worksheet: Therapy.

APPENDICES

The full impact for health care providers of the Health Insurance Portability and Accountability Act of 1996 began to be felt in 2003, when the act's privacy regulations took effect. Many people consider HIPAA's most important provision to be the one about "protected health information," because it requires facilities to take much greater care than before to ensure the information in medical records is kept private. But the real power for patients and their families lies in a short phrase that permits the amendment of medical records. Being able to place your observations directly into the medical records will greatly increase the influence you have over your loved one's care.

Let's say you discover that your loved one has a bedsore, the existence of which is not mentioned in the medical record. By noting this omission with a letter and a photograph that become a permanent part of the record, you can put the nursing home under much greater pressure to respond with appropriate care. Failure to do so would raise a red flag for state and federal auditors and could even result in legal vulnerability. A nursing home has the right to place in the medical record a rebuttal to your amendments, but if you have taken a photograph that clearly illustrates the problem, it would be difficult for the home to refute that evidence. You are required to follow the home's procedures regarding the submission of amendments, but HIPAA (pronounced "hippa") mandates that the home can only refuse them if it asserts that the medical record is accurate and complete.

Were the home to take this approach, you could contact the Health and Human Services Agency to complain about the problem you observed (and documented using the procedures in this book) and the home's failure to include your amendments.

Appendix C contains directions for filing HIPAA-related complaints. The fines for facilities that fail to follow HIPAA regulations are substantial, and the government is intent on making providers adhere to them.

Also included in the Appendices are two sample letters you can use should you need to make an amendment to the medical records. The first letter is to the nursing home administrator. The second is to the medical director or attending physician (sometimes the same person). You will have to insert your particular circumstances, but the samples show you in general how to word a request to amend medical records. Every time you find a problem, document it, photograph it, and make your findings an amendment to the medical records.

In Appendix D we supply some tips for photographing medical conditions. Properly done, photographic documentation can be helpful whether you want to file a complaint or just remind the nursing home's staff that you are monitoring your family member's condition. Bedsores are among the most common problems patients face, so in Appendix E we have provided illustrations of the four stages of bedsores.

Because it can be difficult to keep track of all the participants in your family member's care – among them the nursing home's administrative and medical staffs and outside providers such as an occupational therapist or a speech pathologist – in Appendix F we have provided space for you to list their contact information.

APPENDIX A
Sample Letter to a Nursing Home Administrator

Your Name
Your Address
Your City, State Zip Code

Date

Nursing Home Administrator's Name
Nursing Home Name
Administrator's Address
Administrator's City, State Zip Code

Re: [Patient's Name, Room Number]

Dear [Nursing Home Administrator's Name]:

I am writing to you at this time to confirm our conversation of [date] concerning the failure of your staff to provide adequate nutrition and fluids [or other failure in care] to my [mother, father, or other person]. As you are aware, [she/he] suffers from [state problem, briefly], and requires [solution that has been discussed].

I look forward to receiving a copy of the updated nursing care plan and copies of any documentation of your efforts to assist my [family member]. I am requesting that this letter be considered an amendment to the medical records as provided under HIPAA. If you require that I follow specific procedures to invoke this right under HIPAA, communicate them to me in writing.* Please also confirm in writing that this letter has been made a part of the permanent medical record.

Sincerely,
[Signature]
[Name]

cc: [Name of Director of Nursing], DON
        [Name of Medical Director]
        [Name of Attending Physician if not Medical Director]

Follow the procedure precisely and have your observations and photos placed in the medical record. Confirm this has been done by periodically requesting copies of the record.

APPENDIX B

Sample Letter to a
Medical Director or Attending Physician

Your Name
Your Address
Your City, State Zip Code

Date

Doctor's Name
Doctor's Address
Doctor's City, State Zip Code

Re: [Patient's Name]
Location: [Name of Nursing Home, and Room Number]

Dear Dr. [Name]:

I have reviewed your progress notes for [date] and [date]. The condition of my [mother's, father's, or other person's] skin, especially the grade [stage number] bedsore on the [name area of body], that measures about [length and width in inches or centimeters] has not been addressed. I am writing to request that your progress notes describe this problem and to see a copy of your treatment plan.

As provided by HIPAA, I am requesting that this letter and the attached photograph, dated [date of photo], be entered as an amendment to the medical record.

Sincerely,
[Signature]
[Name]

Cc: [Name of Director of Nursing], DON
      [Name of Nursing Home Administrator], NHA Nursing
       Home Administrator
      [Medical Director's Name if different from
       Attending Physician], Medical Director

APPENDIX C
How to File a HIPAA-Related Complaint

Should you need to file a complaint to make an amendment to the medical record or to initiate one about another HIPAA-related issue, follow the steps below, as outlined in the official literature of the Office for Civil Rights of the U.S. Department of Health and Human Services:

"If you believe that a person, agency or organization covered under the HIPAA Privacy Rule ('a covered entity') violated your (or someone else's) health information privacy rights or committed another violation of the Privacy Rule, you may file a complaint with the Office for Civil Rights (OCR). OCR has authority to receive and investigate complaints against covered entities related to the Privacy Rule. A covered entity is a health plan, health care clearinghouse, and any health care provider who conducts certain health care transactions electronically. . . .

"Complaints to the Office for Civil Rights must: (1) Be filed in writing, either on paper or electronically; (2) name the entity that is the subject of the complaint and describe the acts or omissions believed to be in violation of the applicable requirements of the Privacy Rule; and (3) be filed within 180 days of when you knew that the act or omission complained of occurred. OCR may extend the 180-day period if you can show 'good cause.' Any alleged violation must have occurred on or after April 14, 2003 (on or after April 14, 2004 for small health plans), for OCR to have authority to investigate.

"Anyone can file written complaints with OCR by mail, fax, or email. If you need help filing a complaint or have a question about the complaint form, please call this OCR toll free number: 1-800-368-1019. OCR has ten regional offices, and each regional office covers certain states. You should send your complaint to the appropriate OCR Regional Office, based on the region where the alleged violation took place. Use the OCR Regions list at the end of this Fact Sheet...to help you determine where to send your complaint. Complaints should be sent to the attention of the appropriate OCR Regional Manager."

You can submit your complaint in any written format. The agency recommends that you use the OCR Health Information Privacy Complaint Form, which can be accessed at:

www.memberofthefamily.net/howtofileprivacy.pdf

www.hhs.gov/ocr/hipaa

You can also contact an OCR regional office to obtain a form. If you do not want to use the OCR form, you can submit a written complaint in your own format. If you do so, the OCR recommends that you include the following information:

- Your name, full address, home and work telephone numbers, email address.
- If you are filing a complaint on someone's behalf, also provide the name of the person on whose behalf you are filing.
- Name, full address and phone number of the person, agency, or organization you believe violated your (or someone else's) health information privacy rights or committed another violation of the Privacy Rule.
- Briefly describe what happened. How, when, and why do you believe your (or someone else's) health information privacy rights were violated, or the Privacy Rule otherwise was violated?
- Any other relevant information.
- Please sign your name and date your letter.

- *The following information is optional:*

- Do you need special accommodations for us [the OCR] to communicate with you about this complaint?
- If we cannot reach you directly, is there someone else we can contact to help us reach you?
- Have you filed your complaint somewhere else?

Some family members who have e-mailed our Web site have expressed concern that their complaints will lead to retaliatory action against them or their loved one. The OCR states specifically that "The Privacy Rule, developed under authority of the Health Insurance Portability and Accountability Act of 1996 (HIPAA), prohibits the alleged violating party from taking retaliatory action against anyone for filing a complaint with the Office for Civil Rights. You should notify OCR immediately in the event of any retaliatory action."

OCR Regional Offices

You can e-mail your complaint to OCR at OCRComplaint@hhs.gov or mail or fax it to the appropriate OCR regional office:

Region I – CT, MA, ME, NH, RI, VT
Office for Civil Rights
U.S. Department of Health & Human Services
JFK Federal Building, Room 1875
Boston, MA 02203
Phone: (617) 565-1340; (617) 565-1343 (TDD)
Fax: (617) 565-3809

Region II – NJ, NY, Puerto Rico, U.S. Virgin Islands
Office for Civil Rights
U.S. Department of Health & Human Services
26 Federal Plaza, Suite 3313
New York, NY 10278
Phone: (212) 264-3313; (212) 264-2355 (TDD)
Fax: (212) 264-3039

Region III – DE, DC, MD, PA, VA, WV
Office for Civil Rights
U.S. Department of Health & Human Services
150 South Independence Mall West, Suite 372
Philadelphia, PA 19106
Phone: (215) 861-4441; (215) 861-4440 (TDD)
Fax: (215) 861-4431

Region IV – AL, FL, GA, KY, MS, NC, SC, TN
Office for Civil Rights
U.S. Department of Health & Human Services
61 Forsyth Street, SW, Suite 3B70
Atlanta, GA 30323
Phone: (404) 562-7886; (404) 331-2867 (TDD)
Fax: (404) 562-7881

Region V – IL, IN, MI, MN, OH, WI
Office for Civil Rights
U.S. Department of Health & Human Services
233 North Michigan Avenue, Suite 240
Chicago, IL 60601
Phone: (312) 886-2359; (312) 353-5693 (TDD)
Fax: (312) 886-1807

Region VI – AR, LA, NM, OK, TX
Office for Civil Rights
U.S. Department of Health & Human Services
1301 Young Street, Suite 1169
Dallas, TX 75202
Phone: (214) 767-4056; (214) 767-8940 (TDD)
Fax: (214) 767-0432

Region VII – IA, KS, MO, NE
Office for Civil Rights
U.S. Department of Health & Human Services
601 East 12th Street, Room 248
Kansas City, MO 64106
Phone: (816) 426-7278; (816) 426-7065 (TDD)
Fax: (816) 426-3686

Region VIII – CO, MT, ND, SD, UT, WY
Office for Civil Rights
U.S. Department of Health & Human Services
1961 Stout Street, Room 1426
Denver, CO 80294
Phone: (303) 844-2024; (303) 844-3439 (TDD)
Fax: (303) 844-2025

Region IX – AZ, CA, HI, NV, American Samoa, Guam, and the U.S. Affiliated Pacific Island Jurisdictions
Office for Civil Rights
U.S. Department of Health & Human Services
50 United Nations Plaza, Room 322
San Francisco, CA 94102
Phone: (415) 437-8310; (415) 437-8311 (TDD)
Fax: (415) 437-8329

Region X – AK, ID, OR, WA
Office for Civil Rights
U.S. Department of Health & Human Services
2201 Sixth Avenue, Mail Stop RX-11
Seattle, WA 98121
Phone: (206) 615-2290; (206) 615-2296 (TDD)
Fax: (206) 615-2297

APPENDIX D
Tips on Photographing Medical Conditions

Image composition is a key factor to consider when you photograph medical conditions. The utility of any photo to be used as documentation inevitably comes down to accuracy. The photograph, which will back up any written or oral assertions you might make, must record as precisely as possible what you as an eyewitness have observed.

Don't be squeamish, about privacy or the condition itself. If you are photographing an area that the patient might be embarrassed to have you see, speak to the patient in advance, get his or her permission and make it clear why you are taking photographs. And however difficult it may be to view the condition, keep in mind how you would feel if you had done nothing. The nursing home has every hope that you will not have this kind of record, because a properly taken picture can be worth a thousand words.

Below are some basic guidelines for medical photography:

Use a Good Camera
You don't need professional equipment to document a medical condition, but try to use a camera that you know takes good, clear pictures. Either film or digital photographs will be sufficient. If you do not have access to a good camera, buy two disposable cameras, one that takes close-ups and another with a wider perspective.

Make Sure the Affected Area Is Visible
Clarity is essential. For example, if you are photographing a bedsore, uncover the entire sore and the immediate area around it. Except when you are trying to indicate perspective, compose the shot around the affected area.

Use a Ruler to Show Dimensions
Place a ruler in the photograph to show the dimensions of the affected area. With a bedsore that is not symmetrical, place the ruler so it indicates the longest portion of the sore.

Take Photos from Many Angles
So that there can be no confusion about the condition you are documenting, take photographs from many angles.

Use Flash or Natural Light
Unless you are knowledgeable in the use of filters or the patient has plenty of daylight streaming into his or her room, you are better off using the flash on your camera to light the wound. Turn off any fluorescent lights, as these distort the true colors.

Take Color Photographs
Medical photography is a job for color, not black and white. The color and gradations of color of a wound or sore, for instance, can be crucial information. If the lighting is poor in the room, and you are not using a digital camera, purchase ASA 400 film, especially if you do not have a flash.

Provide Information in the Photograph
The date, the patient's name, the place on the body, and some labeling to indicate head, foot, patient's left and right side can be helpful when the photographs are being viewed. Writing clearly with a black magic marker on a white card "L" or "R" for "left" or "right" or "H" or "F" for "head" or "foot" can be done as needed. To indicate that the photo could not have been taken prior to a certain date, you might consider adding a portion of the local newspaper in one corner of the picture.

Alert the Photo Processing Store's Staff
Let the people at your photo processing store know ahead of time that you have shot medical photographs and that the images may be disturbing. Ask for the prints on paper and on a CD-ROM for archiving.

Review Your Results
If you have shot film, have it developed quickly, but whether you are shooting digitally or with film, review your results as soon as possible. If they do not accurately portray what you have observed, go back and photograph the patient again. (Video cameras can also be used to document a medical condition, but you should turn off the audio. Statements made to reassure or calm your loved one, such as "I'm sure the nurse will be right here" or "Don't worry, they're going to take care of you," can be taken out of context.)

APPENDIX E
Stages of Bedsores

The descriptions of each stage are as defined in the Minimum Data Set, Version 2.0

Stage I: A persistent area of skin redness, without a break in the skin that does not disappear when pressure is relieved.

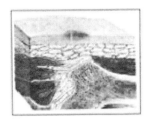

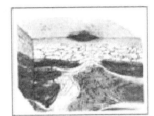

Stage II: A partial thickness loss of skin layers that presents clinically as an abrasion, blister or shallow crater.

Stage III: A full thickness of skin is lost, exposing subcutaneous tissues. It presents as a deep crater with or without undermining adjacent tissues.

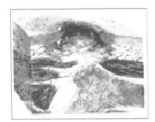

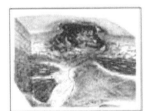

Stage IV: A full thickness of skin and subcutaneous tissue is lost, exposing muscle or bone.

APPENDIX F

Contact Information

Nursing Home

Facility Name: _____

Facility Address: _____

City: _____ State: ____ Zip Code: _____

Telephone Number: (_____) _____

Admissions and Contract Office

Contact Person: _____

Title: _____

Telephone Number: (_____) _____

Billing Office

Contact Person: _____

Title: _____

Telephone Number: (_____) _____

Nursing Home Owner

Manager/President:_____

Corporate Name:_____

Telephone Number: (_____) _____

Providers of Care

Director of Nursing

Name: _____

Telephone Number: (_____) _____

Assistant Director of Nursing

Name: _____

Telephone Number: (_____) _____

Medical Director

Name: _____

Telephone Number: (_____) _____

Custodian of Records

Name: _____

Telephone Number: (_____) _____

HIPAA Compliance Officer

Name: _____

Telephone Number: (_____) _____

Physicians/Medical

Attending Physician

Name: _____

Telephone Number: (_____) _____

Covering Physician

Name: _____

Telephone Number: (_____) _____

Physician's Assistant

Name: _____

Telephone Number: (_____) _____

Nurse Practitioner

Name: _____

Telephone Number: (_____) _____

Dentist

Name: _____

Telephone Number: (_____) _____

Ophthalmologist

Name: _____

Telephone Number: (_____) _____

Podiatrist

Name: _____

Telephone Number: (_____) _____

Mental Health Specialist

Name: _____

Telephone Number: (_____) _____

Other Specialists

Name: _____

Telephone Number: (_____) _____

Name: _____

Telephone Number: (_____) _____

Nursing Services

Registered Nurses

Name: _____

Telephone Number: (_____) _____

Shift: _____

Name: _____

Telephone Number: (_____) _____

Shift: _____

Name: _____

Telephone Number: (_____) _____

Shift: _____

Licensed Practical Nurses

Name: _____

Telephone Number: (_____) _____

Shift: _____

Name: _____

Telephone Number: (_____) _____

Shift: _____

Name: _____

Telephone Number: (_____) _____

Shift: _____

Certified Nursing Aides

Name: _____

Telephone Number: (_____) _____

Shift: _____

Name: _____

Telephone Number: (_____) _____

Shift: _____

Name: _____

Telephone Number: (_____) _____

Shift: _____

Medication Aides

Name: _____

Telephone Number: (_____) _____

Shift: _____

Name: _____

Telephone Number: (_____) _____

Shift: _____

Name: _____

Telephone Number: (_____) _____

Shift: _____

Nursing Aides in Training

Name: _____

Telephone Number: (_____) _____

Shift: _____

Name: _____

Telephone Number: (_____) _____

Shift: _____

Name: _____

Telephone Number: (_____) _____

Shift: _____

Dietary Services

Registered Dietitian

Name: _____

Telephone Number: (_____) _____

Food Service Manager

Name: _____

Telephone Number: (_____) _____

Pharmaceutical Services

Pharmacist

Name: _____

Telephone Number: (_____) _____

Name: _____

Telephone Number: (_____) _____

Therapeutic Services

Occupational Therapist

Name: _____

Telephone Number: (_____) _____

Physical Therapist

Name: _____

Telephone Number: (_____) _____

Speech/Language

Name: _____

Telephone Number: (_____) _____

Activities Professional

Name: _____

Telephone Number: (_____) _____

Social Workers

Name: _____

Telephone Number: (_____) _____

Name: _____

Telephone Number: (_____) _____

Housekeeping Services

Name: _____

Telephone Number: (_____) _____

Providers of Goods

Radiology Services

Name: _____

Telephone Number: (_____) _____

Durable Medical

Name: _____

Telephone Number: (_____) _____

Transportation Services

Name: _____

Telephone Number: (_____) _____

Local Hospital

Name: _____

Telephone Number: (_____) _____

Family and Patient Support Services

Local Ombudsman

Name: _____

Telephone Number: (_____) _____

Family Council Member (if applicable)

Name: _____

Telephone Number: (_____) _____

Resident Council Member (if applicable)

Name: _____

Telephone Number: (_____) _____

Lawyer

Name: _____

Telephone Number: (_____) _____

Clergyman

Name: _____

Telephone Number: (_____) _____

Funeral Director

Name: _____

Telephone Number: (_____) _____

INDEX

About MemberoftheFamily.net

Since 1999, the MemberoftheFamily.net Web site has made its research about more than 16,000 nursing homes available to the public, providing easy-to-understand information from government reports about quality of care and dignity of life in nursing homes. The site lists data about all Medicare- and Medicaid-certified homes in the United States in a report-card format. Color-coded bars reveal at a glance the severity of violations reported over a three-survey period, and the site provides access to data on substantiated complaints about individual homes. Thousands of users visit the Web site, www.memberofthefamily.net, each month. The site's National Watch List provides details from currently available surveys and includes homes with citations for actions and deficiencies that resulted in actual harm or immediate jeopardy to their residents.

MemberoftheFamily.net receives numerous letters of support each week from families and individuals. Administrators also contact the site, sometimes to say thanks for helping to improve the industry and other times to discuss or question reported survey results. Feedback from site users indicates that the information they access helps them to understand the nursing home rating system, identify homes that are consistently found to be providing substandard care, and protect their loved ones from peril.

❑ ❑ ❑

Danger Zone is the first MemberoftheFamily.net LifeGuide®. To order copies of *Danger Zone* or to contact the book's authors, write to MemberoftheFamily.net, 670 Ritchie Highway, Severna Park, MD 21146, or log onto www.memberofthefamily.net. *Danger Zone* is available at a special discount for bulk purchases for individuals or organizations.

About the Authors

Edward C. Watters III, M.D.

Edward C. "Terry" Watters III, M.D., the cofounder of MemberoftheFamily.net, graduated in 1981 from the University of Maryland School of Medicine. Following the completion of his first-year residency training in internal medicine at Mercy Hospital in Baltimore, Maryland, he returned to the University of Maryland Hospital to complete his residency in ophthalmology in 1985. Since that time he has served as a consulting ophthalmologist to six nursing homes, and since the mid-1990s he has served as a physician advisor to the State of Maryland Department of Health and Mental Hygiene. In this role he has developed numerous software programs to analyze health-care data. The results of many of these studies have influenced health-care policy, particularly regarding the monitoring of quality, access, and finances in the state Medicaid Program. Dr. Watters, who has been recognized numerous times by the Department of Health and Mental Hygiene for his outstanding contributions, is a member of the teaching staff of the University of Maryland School of Medicine and also maintains an active medical and surgical practice.

Dennis R. Steele

Dennis R. Steele, the cofounder of MemberoftheFamily.net, graduated from Towson University in 1975, where he majored in philosophy, and continued his graduate studies in business at Johns Hopkins University. He is an executive with a Baltimore corporation, where he has played a key role in establishing computer systems and migrating data to newer platforms. Bringing a nonmedical perspective to MemberoftheFamily.net, he constructed and maintains the Web site on which the group posts its data about nursing homes. He has appeared on televised panel discussions about nursing home care on behalf of MemberoftheFamily.net and has extensively researched the business side of the industry.

The authors are grateful for the guidance of our editor, Danny Mangin, who helped us focus on the core issues of this complex topic.

Danger Zone
Unlock the Secrets of Nursing Home Medical Records and Protect Your Loved One

ORDER FORM

Name _____

Shipping address _____

City _____
State _____ Zip _____

Phone _____
E-mail _____
(in case we need to contact you about your order)

Single copy: $14.95; 10 or more copies: $13.95 each
Price includes standard shipping when you order directly from MemberoftheFamily.net.
Overnight delivery additional. Maryland State residents add 5% sales tax.

_____ # of copies X _____ price = order total $ _____

TO ORDER BY PHONE

Call (410) 421-9100 Monday – Friday 9:00 a.m. – 4:00 p.m. EST/DST
Please have credit card information available when you call.

TO ORDER BY FAX OR MAIL

_____ Charge to MasterCard   Acct. # _____ Exp.___ /___

_____ Charge to VISA   Acct. # _____ Exp.___ /___

Name on card _____
Credit card billing address if different from shipping address:

Address _____
City _____
State _____ Zip _____

Signature _____

_____ To order by fax, send form to our secure fax: **410-544-4463**

_____ To order by mail, fill out credit card form above (or enclose check) and send to:

MemberoftheFamily.net
670 Ritchie Highway
Severna Park, MD 21146